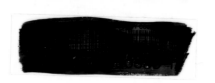

Cross Training for Fitness

Matt Brzycki

Coordinator of Health Fitness, Strength and Conditioning

Princeton University

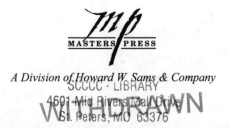

MP
MASTERS PRESS

A Division of Howard W. Sams & Company

Published by Masters Press
A Division of Howard W. Sams & Company
2647 Waterfront Pkwy E. Dr, Suite 100, Indianapolis, IN 46214

97 98 99 00 01 02   10 9 8 7 6 5 4 3 2 1

Library of Congress Cataloging-in-Publication Data
Brzycki, Matt.
    Cross Training for Fitness / Matt Brzycki.
        p.   cm.
    Includes bibliographical references (p.).
    ISBN 1-57028-107-6 (trade paper)
    1. Physical fitness. 2. Exercise. 3. Physical education and
training. I. Title.
GV481.B79 1997   96-52668
613.7'1--dc21   CIP

DEDICATION

This book is dedicated to my wife, Alicia, and our child.

Table of Contents

ACKNOWLEDGEMENTS

Personal thanks to Tony Alexander, Marcus Amick, Rich Burton, Andy Foltiny, Ken Mannie, Wayne Meyer, Sasha Ruiz, Brendan Tierney, Trevor Tierney, Greg Williams and Shane Woolf for volunteering their time as book models.

Grateful appreciation to Masters Press including Tom Bast (publisher), Holly Kondras (managing editor), Phil Velikan (designer), and Bryan Banschbach (proofreader) and other staff members who helped make this project a reality.

Special recognition to the equipment manufacturers who supplied pictures from their files including Concept II, Incorporated; Heart Rate, Incorporated; Nautilus International; Quinton Fitness Equipment; and StairMaster Sports/ Medical Products, Incorporated.

A final round of thanks to the Office of Athletic Communications at Princeton University for once again allowing me unrestricted access to their photographs.

1

The Value of Cross Training

The so-called fitness boom of the 1970s has proven to be a bit of a misnomer. By definition, a "boom" means a sudden, rapid expansion or increase in importance. While fitness may have experienced its boom in the 1970s, fitness has enjoyed a continued and growing increase in importance, acceptance and popularity that appears to be unending. In retrospect, the "fitness boom" may be more aptly described as a "fitness trend."

As the popularity of fitness has grown, so has the interest in being involved in varied conditioning activities. In recent years, the term "cross training" — or "cross conditioning" — has become a buzzword among fitness enthusiasts everywhere. In reality, however, cross training has actually been practiced for a number of years — though it has been done under the unsophisticated and informal guise of "variety in exercise." The affiliation of cross training with varied activities is exemplified by cross-training shoes — or "Cross Trainers" — which are essentially multi-purpose footwear.

The first application of cross-training methods may have been by competitive triathletes. These athletes are required to be highly proficient at three different types of physical efforts: swimming, outdoor cycling and running. Their need for varied conditioning activities may very well have been the stimulus for the current widespread appeal and appreciation of cross training by recreational fitness enthusiasts.

ADVANTAGES OF CROSS TRAINING

There are many advantages of cross training for fitness. Perhaps its biggest benefit is that it provides you with variety in your workouts. In fact, the cornerstone of cross training is that it promotes the use of different activities.

A fitness program that includes assorted activities is very appealing and reduces the probability that you'll become bored from sheer monotony. A program that isn't boring or monotonous also increases the likelihood that you'll continue with your quest for improved fitness.

Frequently changing your activities is an excellent way to overcome plateaus in your training. Remember, the ultimate purpose of cross training is to improve your level of fitness by applying a progressively greater workload — or an "overload" — on your circulatory, respiratory and musculoskeletal systems. The activities you perform aren't as critical as other program variables such as the intensity of your workout and the duration of your activity. So, it doesn't really matter whether you pedal a stationary cycle during one workout and use a stair climber during the next — as long as the demands you've placed on your physiological systems are increasingly more challenging.

Cross training can also allow you to continue exercising despite an injury which might otherwise prohibit you from training. For example, it's highly unlikely that you'd be able to run in a pain-free fashion with shin splints. However, it's more than likely that you'd be able to exercise with little or no discomfort by performing another cross-training activity that is non-weightbearing — such as swimming or cycling.

In addition, cross training reduces your risk of repetitive-stress injuries which may occur from performing a physically stressful activity over and over again for long periods of time. By periodically substituting one or more comparable cross-training activity, you can still exercise the same muscles but in a different and less stressful manner.

THE BENEFITS OF REGULAR EXERCISE

Cross training for fitness provides all of the benefits associated with regular physical activity. Clearly, those who exercise regularly receive many specific psychological, physiological and physical rewards.

From a psychological standpoint, regular exercise relieves stress and anxiety, improves mood and prevents depression. Habitual physical activity also improves general well-being, increases self-esteem and nurtures a positive body image. Regular physical activity improves physical appearance which also contributes to psychological satisfaction. Finally, regular exercise averts mental burnout and prevents discouragement.

Right: The Cornerstone of cross training is that it promotes the use of different activities. (photo provided by Quinton Fitness Equipment)

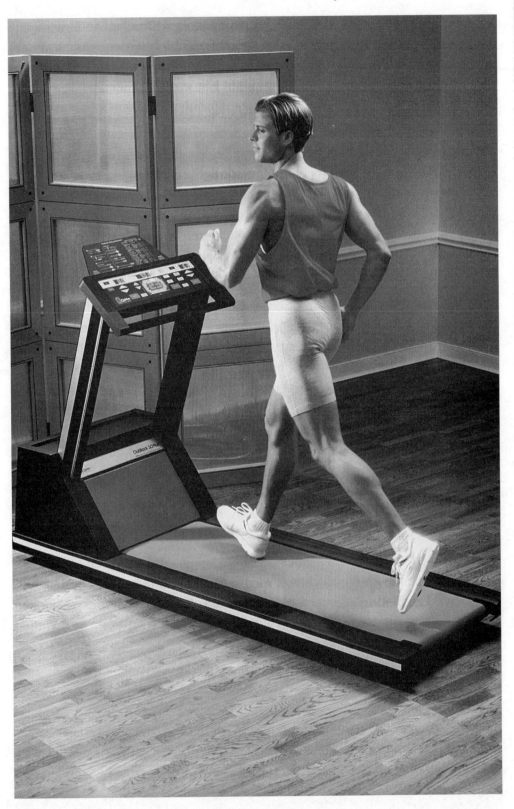

Exercise also provides a wide range of physiological benefits. An individual who exercises on a regular basis has a lower resting heart rate than a sedentary counterpart. As fitness levels improve, a person's heart rate recovers faster from exercise and returns to its resting level more quickly.

Being fit makes it easier for the average person to perform everyday activities such as climbing stairs, mowing grass and carrying groceries. From an athletic perspective, a highly conditioned person can work at greater levels of intensity for longer periods of time at a lower heart rate than someone who is less conditioned. This "conditioning advantage" means that a person who is involved in a competitive sport or activity won't have to expend as much energy as an opponent and will be able to perform activities with less visible effort. Besides increasing an athlete's performance potential, routine exercise also reduces an athlete's injury potential.

Exercising on a regular basis reduces your risk of Coronary Heart Disease (CHD) which is the leading cause of premature death in the United States. Numerous risk factors associated with CHD have been identified including lack of activity, obesity, elevated cholesterol levels and hypertension (i.e., high blood pressure). Habitual exercise has a positive impact on several risk factors. For instance, engaging in a fitness program increases your activity levels and — if done in conjunction with wise nutritional planning — helps you attain and maintain an acceptable percentage of body fat and/or bodyweight. Regular exercise has been found to increase high-density lipoprotein or HDL (i.e., the "good" cholesterol). Individuals with higher levels of HDL are less prone to CHD. Lastly, regular physical activity lowers resting blood pressure.

Those who exercise routinely have increased elasticity in their arteries and a reduced tendency for blood clots to form where the arteries have narrowed. These biological adaptations lower the risk of a stroke. Additionally, being active reduces the risk of disease (such as colon cancer), improves general health and the quality of life.

Regular physical activity offers protection against non-insulin dependent diabetes mellitus. Exercising regularly also helps regulate the blood glucose levels of diabetic individuals. Exercise increases insulin sensitivity and, therefore, is part of the treatment program for diabetics whose blood sugar is well-controlled. (It is recommended that diabetics consult a physician before beginning an exercise program.)

There are several benefits from exercising regularly that are specific to older individuals. In general, performing physical activity on a regular basis delays the loss of strength and lean body mass that usually accompanies the aging process. Older individuals who exercise also experience an increase in bone density which helps combat the adverse effects of osteoporosis.

A PRODUCTIVE CHOICE

People are continually searching for new and improved methods of achieving their fitness goals. For various reasons, growing numbers of individuals are adopting cross training as their method of choice. Clearly, one of the best ways to reach your physical potential is by cross training for fitness.

2

Basic Anatomy and Muscular Function

Cross training is a series of movements that are made by your musculoskeletal system. To obtain a better appreciation of these musculoskeletal movements, it's necessary to understand some basic anatomy and muscular function.

Your body is basically a system of levers. Movement of these levers — your bones — is produced by your muscles, which are anchored to your bones by tendons. (Tendons link muscle to bone; ligaments link bone to bone.) Perhaps the most well-known and noticeable tendon in your body is your Achilles tendon which fastens your calf muscles to your heel bone.

MUSCLE: TYPES AND STRUCTURE

There are three different types of muscle tissue: cardiac, smooth and skeletal. Cardiac muscle makes up most of your heart wall, smooth muscle is found in the walls of your blood vessels and skeletal muscle acts across your joints to produce movement.

Your muscles are made up of numerous muscle fibers which, in turn, are made up of many myofibrils. (To get an idea of this arrangement, picture a telephone cable containing hundreds of wires.) Myofibrils contain two contractile protein filaments — the thin actin and the thicker myosin — which lie parallel to one another. Muscular contractions occur at this level.

MUSCLE CONTRACTIONS

Contraction refers to the process of a muscle generating a force. The force exerted by a contracting muscle on an object is known as the muscle tension; the force exerted by the weight of an object on a muscle is known as the load. Therefore, muscle tension and load are opposing forces.

There are three types of muscle contractions: concentric, eccentric and isometric. Although isometric contractions rarely occur during cross-training activities, both concentric and eccentric contractions take place regularly.

A concentric muscle contraction is one in which a muscle shortens against a load. The movement of the resistance is done in a direction away from the earth or opposite the direction of gravity. Examples of concentric contractions are raising a weight, rising from a squat position or running uphill. In a concentric muscle contraction, muscular tension is greater than the external load. Since the mechanical work is positive, a concentric muscle contraction is sometimes referred to as the positive phase of a movement.

An eccentric muscular contraction occurs when a muscle lengthens against a load. The movement of the resistance is done in a direction toward the earth or in the direction of gravity. Examples of eccentric contractions are lowering a weight, descending into a squat position or running downhill. In an eccentric muscle contraction, muscular tension is less than the external load. Because the mechanical work is negative, an eccentric contraction is typically referred to as the negative phase of a movement.

Finally, an isometric (or static) contraction is one in which the contractile component of a muscle shortens while the elastic connective tissue lengthens by the same amount, thereby producing no change in the overall muscle-tendon length. An example of an isometric contraction would be holding a weight in a static position, maintaining a squat position or exerting tension against an immovable object. Since no movement takes place during an isometric muscle contraction, the mechanical work is zero. (Of course, energy must be provided in order to produce an isometric muscle contraction. Although there is no mechanical work performed, there is metabolic work.)

THE SLIDING FILAMENT THEORY

Movement of your musculoskeletal system is produced by contraction of your muscles. The most widely accepted theory of explaining muscular contraction is the Sliding Filament Theory. As the name of this theory implies, one set of proteinous filaments is thought to slide over the other and overlap (like pistons in a sleeve), thereby shortening the muscle. Here's how: The myosin filaments have tiny protein projections in the shape of globular heads, which extend toward the actin filaments. During a concentric muscular contraction, it's believed that these projections — or "crossbridges" — bind to the actin filament and then swivel in a ratchetlike fashion — much like oars in a boat — in such a way that it pulls the actin over the myosin filament. The crossbridges then uncouple from the actin, pivot, reattach and repeat the cycle. Thus, this process can be summed up as "attach-rotate-detach-rotate." A single myosin crossbridge may attach and detach with an actin filament hundreds of times in the course of a single muscular contraction (e.g., during one repetition of an exercise). This process occurs along the entire myofibril and among all the myofibrils of a muscle fiber. However, the crossbridges do not attach-rotate-detach-rotate at the same time since this would result in a series of jerks rather than a smooth movement.

COMMON JOINT MOVEMENTS

Several terms are frequently used in exercise jargon to describe various joint movements. Familiarity with these terms will assist you in understanding the function of most muscles.

Flexion is a decrease in the angle between two bones. The opposite of flexion is extension, which is an increase in the angle between two bones. Abduction refers to movement of a limb away from the midline of the body. Conversely, adduction is movement of a limb toward the midline of the body. Finally, rotation is turning about the vertical axis of a bone.

THE MAJOR MUSCLES

Incredible as it may seem, there are more than 600 muscles in the human body — and about six billion muscle fibers. In fact, each one of your forearms is made up of 19 separate muscles with such exotic-sounding names as "extensor carpi radialis brevis" and "flexor digitorum superficialis." It's well beyond the scope and purpose of this book to discuss your muscles in such great detail. Instead, this chapter only focuses on your major muscle groups.

The major muscle groups described are the hips, legs, upper torso, arms, neck, abdominals and lower back. These seven major muscle groups are further subdivided into their most important components. Brief notes on the location and function of each muscle are given along with anatomical terminology that is generally accepted in discussions of exercise.

Hips

Buttocks. The buttocks muscles are the largest and strongest muscles in your body. Your buttocks are composed of three main muscle groups: the gluteus maximus, the gluteus medius and the gluteus minimus. The primary function of the gluteus maximus is hip extension (driving your upper leg backward); the main function of the gluteus medius and the gluteus minimus is hip abduction (spreading your legs apart). The "glutes" are important muscles used in walking, running, jumping and stair-climbing activities.

Adductors. The adductor group is composed of five muscles that are located throughout your inner thigh: the gracilis, the pectineus, the adductor longus, the adductor brevis and the adductor magnus (which is the largest of these five muscles). The muscles of your inner thigh are used during adduction of your hip (bringing your legs together).

Iliopsoas. This is a collective term for the two primary muscles of your front hip area: the iliacus and the psoas. The main function of the iliopsoas is to flex your hip (bring your knee to your chest). Your iliopsoas plays a major role in many cross-training activities — especially those that involve lifting your knees such as when you walk or run. The iliacus and the psoas are sometimes considered with the muscles of the abdomen.

Legs

Hamstrings. The "hams" are located on the backside of your upper leg and actually include three separate muscles: the semimembranosus, the semitendinosus and the biceps femoris. Together, these muscles are involved in flexing your lower leg around your knee joint (bringing your heel toward your hip) and in hip extension. Your hamstrings are used during virtually all running and jumping activities. Unfortunately, the muscle is very susceptible to pulls and tears. Strong hamstrings are necessary to balance the effects of the powerful quadricep muscles.

Quadriceps. The "quads" are the most important muscles on the front part of your thigh. As the name suggests, your quadriceps are made up of four muscles. The vastus lateralis is located on the outside of your thigh; the vastus medialis resides on the inner (medial) side of your thigh above your patella (the kneecap); between these two thigh muscles is the vastus intermedius; and finally, laying on top of the vastus intermedius is the rectus femoris. The main function of the quads is extending (or straightening) your lower leg at the knee joint. Your quads are involved in walking, running, cycling, kicking, jumping and stair-climbing activities.

Calves. Your calves are made up of two important muscles — the gastrocnemius (or "gastroc") and the soleus — which are located on the backside of your lower leg. Sometimes these two muscles are jointly referred to as the "triceps surae" or, more simply, the "gastroc-soleus." Your soleus actually resides underneath your gastroc and is used primarily when your knee is bent at 90 degrees or more (e.g., in the seated position). The calves are involved when your foot is extended at your ankle (or when rising up on your toes). This action is known as plantar flexion. The calves play a major role in running and jumping activities.

Dorsi Flexors. The front part of your lower leg contains four muscles that are sometimes simply referred to as the "dorsi flexors." The largest of these muscles is the tibialis anterior. The dorsi flexors are primarily used in flexing your foot toward your knee and are involved when cycling with toe clips. It is critical to strengthen the dorsi flexors as a safeguard against shin splints.

Upper Torso

Chest. The major muscle surrounding your chest area is the pectoralis major. It is thick, flat and fan-shaped and is the most superficial muscle of your chest wall. The pectoralis minor is a thin, flat triangular muscle that is positioned beneath your pectoralis major. The "pecs" pull your upper arm down and across your body. Like most of the upper-torso muscles, your pecs are involved in throwing and pushing movements.

Upper Back. The latissimus dorsi is the long, broad muscle that comprises most of your upper back. The "lats" are the largest muscles in your upper body. Their primary function is to pull your upper arm backward and downward. The latissimus dorsi is particularly important in pulling movements and climbing skills. In addition, developing the latissimus dorsi is necessary to provide muscular balance between your upper back and your chest areas.

Shoulders. Your shoulders are made up of 11 muscles of which the deltoids are the most important. Your "delts" are actually composed of three separate parts or "heads." The anterior deltoid is found on the front of your shoulder and is used when raising your upper arm forward; the middle deltoid is found on the side of your shoulder and is involved when your upper arm is lifted sideways (away from the body); the posterior deltoid resides on the back of your shoulder and draws your upper arm backward. Several other deep muscles of the shoulder are sometimes referred to as the "internal rotators" (the subscapularis and the teres major) and the "external rotators" (the infraspinatus and the teres minor). In addition to performing rotation, these muscles are also largely responsible for maintaining the integrity of your shoulder joint and in preventing shoulder impingement. Along with the muscles of the pectoral region, strong shoulders are a vital part of swimming, throwing skills and pushing movements.

Arms

Biceps. The biceps brachii is the prominent muscle on the front part of your upper arm. It causes your arm to flex (or bend) at your elbow. As the name suggests, the biceps has two separate parts or "heads." The separation can sometimes be seen as a groove on a well-developed arm when the biceps are fully flexed. Your biceps assist your upper-torso muscles — especially your lats — in pulling movements and climbing skills.

Triceps. The triceps brachii is a horseshoe-shaped muscle located on the backside of your upper arm. This muscle has three distinct heads — the long, the lateral and the medial. The primary function of your triceps is to extend (or straighten) your arm at your elbow. Your triceps assist your upper-torso muscles in throwing skills and pushing movements.

Forearms. As stated earlier, your forearm is made up of 19 different muscles. These muscles may be divided into two groups on the basis of their position and functions. The anterior group on the front part of your forearm causes flexion and pronation (turning your palm downward); the posterior group on the back part of your forearm causes extension and supination (turning your palm upward). Your forearms effect your wrists and hands, which are important in pulling movements, climbing skills and tasks that involve gripping.

Neck

Neck Flexors. The muscles on the front part of your neck can be collectively referred to as the "neck flexors." A major neck flexor is your sternocleido-mastoideus. This muscle has two heads — one located on each side of your neck — which start behind your ears and run down to your sternum (breastbone) and clavicles (collarbones). When both sides of the sternocleido-mastoideus contract at the same time, your head is flexed toward your chest; when one side acts singly, your head is brought laterally toward your shoulder or is rotated to the side.

Neck Extensors. The back portion of your neck contains several muscles that can simply be referred to as the "neck extensors." The neck extensors are mainly used to extend your head backward.

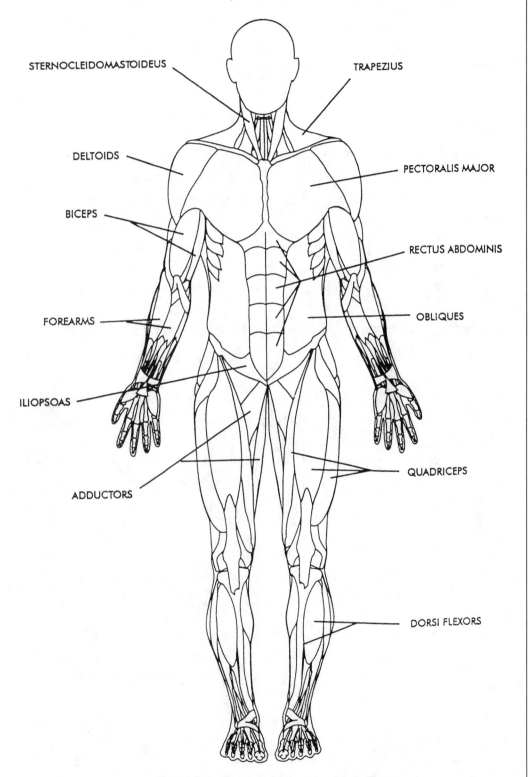

STERNOCLEIDOMASTOIDEUS

TRAPEZIUS

DELTOIDS

PECTORALIS MAJOR

BICEPS

RECTUS ABDOMINIS

FOREARMS

OBLIQUES

ILIOPSOAS

QUADRICEPS

ADDUCTORS

DORSI FLEXORS

Figure 2.1: Anterior view of the muscles of the body

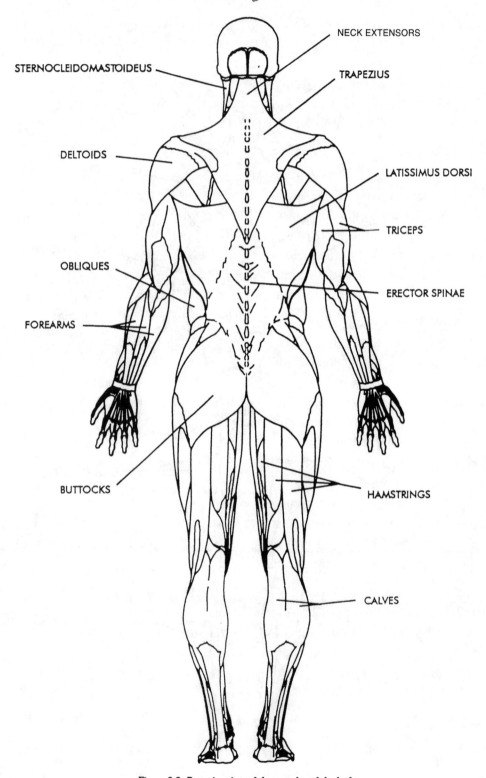

Figure 2.2: Posterior view of the muscles of the body

Trapezius. The trapezius is a kite-shaped (or trapezoid-shaped) muscle that covers the uppermost region of your back and the posterior section of your neck. The primary functions of your "traps" are to elevate your shoulders (as in shrugging), to adduct your scapulae (pinch your shoulder blades together) and to extend your head backward. The trapezius is often considered part of the shoulder musculature.

Abdominals

Rectus Abdominis. This long, narrow muscle extends vertically across the front of your abdomen from the lower rim of your rib cage to your pelvis. Its main function is to pull your torso toward your lower body. The fibers of this muscle are interrupted along their course by three horizontal fibrous bands, which give rise to the phrase "washboard abs" when describing an especially well-developed abdomen. The rectus abdominis helps to control your breathing and plays a major role in forced expiration during intense exercise.

Obliques. The external and internal obliques lie on both sides of your waist. The external oblique is a broad muscle whose fibers form a V across the front of your abdominal area, extending diagonally downward from your lower ribs to your pubic bone. The main function of this muscle is to bend your upper torso to the same side and to rotate your torso to the opposite side. The internal obliques lie immediately under your external obliques on both sides of your abdomen. The fibers of your internal obliques form an inverted V along the front of your abdominal wall, extending diagonally upward from your pubic bone to your ribs. The internal obliques bend your upper body to the same side and turn your torso to the same side. Your obliques are used in movements in which your upper torso twists or rotates. The internal and external obliques are also active during expiration and inspiration, respectively.

Transversus Abdominis. The transversus abdominis is the innermost layer of your abdominal musculature. The fibers of this muscle run horizontally across your abdomen. The primary function of the transversus abdominis is to constrict your abdomen. This muscle is also involved in forced expiration and in control of your breathing.

Lower Back

Erector Spinae. The "spinal erectors" make up the main muscle group in your lower back. Their primary purpose is to extend (or straighten) your upper torso from a bent-over position. However, the erector spinae also assists in bending your torso laterally and in rotating your torso. Low-back pain is one of the most common and costly medical problems today. It has been estimated that 80 percent of the world's population will experience low-back pain sometime in their lives with annual costs of more than $50 billion. Insufficient strength seems to be a factor related to low-back pain.

3
The Physiology of Cross Training

One of the most remarkable organisms on our planet is the human body. It's important for you to understand how your body produces and utilizes energy during your cross-training activities. Familiarity with your various metabolic systems will also help you understand how the processes effect your physical performance.

ADENOSINE TRIPHOSPHATE

The energy liberated during the breakdown of food is used to make a chemical compound called adenosine triphosphate, or more simply, ATP. This compound is stored in most living cells — particularly muscle cells — and has an extremely high energy yield. The structure of ATP consists of an adenosine component that is bonded to three chemically-important phosphate groups. The energy from ATP is not necessarily in its chemical make-up, but in the so-called high-energy phosphate bonds which hold the compound together. When one of the phosphate bonds is broken — or removed from the rest of the molecule — energy is released and adenosine diphosphate (ADP) plus inorganic phosphate are formed. The energy liberated during the breakdown of ATP is your primary — and immediate — source of energy used to perform muscular work.

YOUR ENERGY SYSTEMS

In order to exercise for prolonged periods of time, a constant supply of ATP must be made available to your muscle cells. Unfortunately, your muscle cells can only store a limited amount of ATP. As such, your cells must be capable of resynthesizing — or rebuilding — ATP from ADP and inorganic phosphate.

A typical ATP molecule may exist for only a few seconds before its bonds are broken and energy is released. The ADP formed by this chemical event is rapidly remade into ATP. Interestingly, energy is also required to resynthesize ATP. In fact, all of your energy systems have one common and primary purpose: to reconstruct ATP in order to supply energy so that your muscles can perform physical work.

The process by which ATP is reassembled involves the interaction of three different series of chemical reactions. Two of these do not require the presence of oxygen and are termed "anaerobic"; the other series of reactions can only operate in the existence of oxygen and is labeled "aerobic." Your two anaerobic energy systems are the ATP-PC System and Anaerobic Glycolysis; your aerobic source is known as the Aerobic System.

The ATP-PC System

In your ATP-PC (or Phosphagen) System, the energy used to rebuild ATP comes from the breakdown of a chemical compound known as phosphocreatine or, more simply, PC. Like ATP, PC is stored in your muscle cells and has a rather high energy yield. Since ATP and PC both contain phosphate groups, they are collectively referred to as "phosphagens." Similar to ATP, PC releases a large amount of energy when its phosphate group is removed. (The end-products of this breakdown are creatine and inorganic phosphate.) The energy yielded by this process is immediately available and is used to reconstruct ATP. In fact, as quickly as ATP is broken down during muscular efforts, it is continuously re-manufactured by the energy released from the breakdown of PC. Ironically, PC can only be rebuilt from the energy released by the breakdown of ATP.

The phosphagen stores in your working muscles — that is, your ATP and PC pools — would probably be spent after an all-out exertion lasting about a handful of seconds. If you're in reasonably good condition, this equates to sprinting roughly 50 yards or swimming about 10 yards at breakneck speed. So, the total amount of ATP energy available from your Phosphagen System is very limited. Obviously, the usefulness of your stored phosphagens lies in their rapid availability rather than their quantity. Fast, powerful movements — such as sprinting and jumping — could not be performed without this metabolic system. It's no surprise then that your ATP-PC System is the predominant energetic pathway for exercise or efforts of very high intensity and brief duration — less than about 30 seconds.

Right: Fast, powerful movements — such as sprinting and jumping — could not be performed without your ATP-PC System. (Photo by David Coyle)

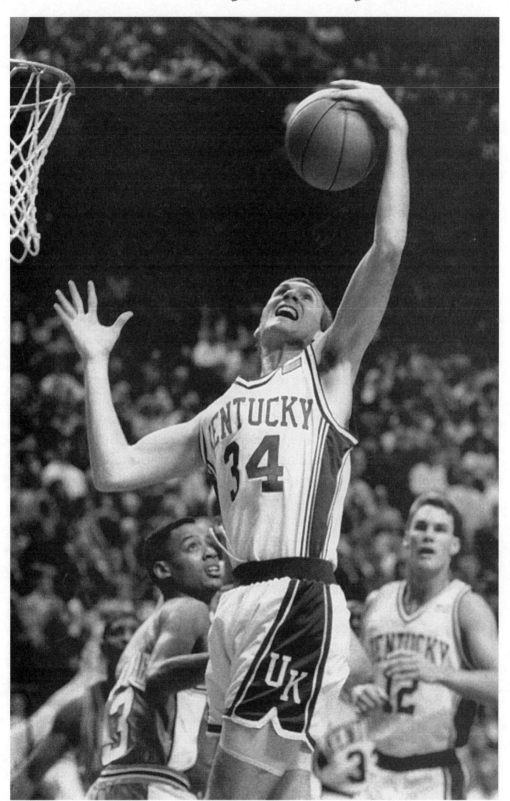

Anaerobic Glycolysis

In your body, carbohydrates are converted to glucose — or "blood sugar" — which can either be instantly utilized in that form or stored as glycogen in your liver and muscles for later use. The term "glycolysis" means "to break down glycogen" and, as noted earlier, "anaerobic" basically means "without oxygen." Therefore, Anaerobic Glycolysis literally refers to the breakdown of glycogen in the absence of oxygen. When glycogen is broken down, energy is released and is used to reassemble ATP. However, a complete breakdown of glycogen requires oxygen. Since oxygen isn't required during Anaerobic Glycolysis, the breakdown of glycogen is only partial and forms pyruvic acid as a by-product. Pyruvic acid is subsequently converted into a substance called "lactic acid" (or "lactate") — which is why Anaerobic Glycolysis is often referred to as the "Lactic Acid System."

When you burn a log you are always left with ash as a waste product. Similarly, lactic acid is the glycolytic ash of this anaerobic pathway. The point at which lactic acid first begins to appear in your blood is known as your "anaerobic threshold." When lactic acid enters your blood at a greater rate than it is removed, there is a rise in the concentration of lactic acid in your blood. High concentrations of lactic acid can irritate your nerve endings and cause pain. The accumulation of lactate is also believed to cause excessive breathing, feelings of fatigue and heaviness in the muscles. Because it is a fatiguing by-product, lactic acid essentially acts as a performance inhibitor during Anaerobic Glycolysis. In fact, your muscles and blood can only tolerate about 2.0 - 2.5 ounces of lactic acid before fatigue occurs. (Some lactic acid is formed under resting conditions but it doesn't accumulate because the rate of production equals the rate of removal.)

Anaerobic Glycolysis — with a helping hand from your ATP-PC System — is responsible for supplying ATP for all maximal efforts that last between approximately 30 - 90 seconds. For those with an acceptable level of fitness, this time-frame correlates to sprinting a distance of roughly 220 - 440 yards. Therefore, the first minute or two of exercise depends upon your ability to replenish ATP without the use of oxygen. The resynthesis of ATP is quite rapid but — without the presence of oxygen — is somewhat limited.

The Aerobic System

Essentially, we have an unlimited supply of oxygen available. Indeed, it is everywhere around us. However, the amount of energy that can be produced with the use of oxygen is determined by the efficiency of your Aerobic System.

During exercise, your Aerobic System is the last process in your chemical chain-of-command for energy production. In the Aerobic System, glycogen is once again broken down to release energy that is used to rebuild ATP — which is why this system is sometimes called "Aerobic Glycolysis." Because oxygen is used in this process, the breakdown of glycogen is complete. Relative to your anaerobic systems, your Aerobic System can operate for a longer duration because no fatiguing by-products — such as lactic acid — are formed in the presence of oxygen. Rather than form lactic acid from pyruvic acid, this particular system converts pyruvic acid into two end-products: carbon dioxide and water. However, carbon dioxide is continually removed by the blood and transported to the lungs where it is exhaled; water is either used in the cell or excreted in the urine. So, glycolytic reactions occur in both the aerobic and anaerobic domains — the difference is that lactic acid isn't formed when sufficient oxygen is available. Another feature of your Aerobic System is that it can also break down both carbohydrates and fats to liberate energy for the reconstruction of ATP, while anaerobically only carbohydrates can be used. (Protein — the third macronutrient — isn't normally used as a source of energy.)

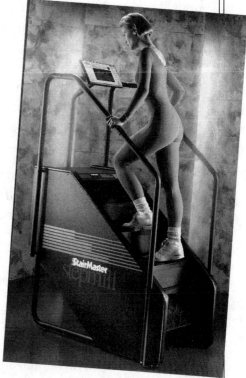

The process of rebuilding ATP aerobically occurs in specialized areas of your muscle cells called mitochondria. These areas produce such a large amount of energy that the mitochondria are often referred to as the "powerhouse" of the cell. Muscle cells are usually very rich with mitochondria. In particular, an abundance of mitochondria is found in cardiac muscle and slow-twitch muscle fibers.

Your Aerobic System becomes the primary energetic pathway once your anaerobic systems are unable to keep up with the metabolic demands of the activity and lactic acid begins to accumulate. Activities that are between 1.5 - 3.0 minutes in duration are the shared responsibility of Anaerobic Glycolysis and the Aerobic System. For the most part, your Aerobic System becomes the

Above: Your Aerobic System becomes the primary source of energy after roughly three minutes of continuous exertion. (photo provided by StairMaster Sports/Medical Products, Inc.)

principal source of energy after roughly three minutes of continuous exertion which would correlate to a running distance beyond about one-half mile. (Research suggests that at least 10 - 15 minutes of continuous activity is usually needed for you to obtain aerobic benefits. For those in reasonably good condition, this equates to a distance of roughly 1.5 miles.) The longer the duration of exercise, the greater the importance of your Aerobic System. Interestingly, your Aerobic System is also the preferred energetic pathway under resting conditions.

A major advantage of your Aerobic System is that it produces relatively large amounts of energy. However, the Aerobic System is a time-consuming process due to the transport and delivery of oxygen. Therefore, this system cannot produce energy rapidly enough to meet the demands of short-term, high-intensity movements such as jumping and sprinting.

THE ENERGY CONTINUUM

The need for a particular energy system is determined by the time and intensity requirements of a specific activity. At one end of the so-called energy continuum is your anaerobic ATP-PC System which is the dominant energy pathway for short-term, high-intensity efforts; at the other end of the scale is your Aerobic System which is the principal energy pathway for long-term, low-intensity work. In between these two extremes of the continuum, the vast majority of your energy is supplied by Anaerobic Glycolysis. Also in the middle of the continuum are many sports and cross-training activities which require a mixture of both your anaerobic and aerobic pathways, such as running 440 - 880 yards, rowing 400 - 800 yards, swimming 100 - 200 yards, wrestling 2- or 3- minute periods and boxing 3-minute rounds.

Your body does not exclusively choose one metabolic pathway over another — your exercising muscles simply use whatever energy source is readily available to meet the physiological demands. Generally, your body selects the most efficient metabolic pathway to maximize ATP resynthesis and to minimize lactic acid accumulation.

Your level of blood lactate is an excellent indicator of which energy system you mainly relied upon during your effort. A high level of blood lactate indicates that Anaerobic Glycolysis was your primary energetic system; a low level of blood lactate means that your Aerobic System was your dominant energetic system.

Although one of your three metabolic pathways may serve as the primary source of energy for a given activity, all three pathways contribute to the supply of ATP that is required to perform most activities. Stated otherwise, both anaerobic and aerobic pathways contribute some ATP during physical performance with one system generally contributing more. For example, tennis is primarily anaerobic because it consists largely of a series of brief, all-out efforts such as sprinting short distances, hitting serves, returning shots and so on. However, tennis also has an aerobic component since the anaerobic movements are required over a fairly long period of time. There-fore, energy is needed from both the anaerobic and aerobic systems. In fact, a blend of all energetic pathways is the most likely scenario for the majority of sports and activities.

As the time of an activity increases, the continuum shifts away from anaero-bic work toward aerobic work. It should also be noted that your energy systems operate in phases on a progressive scale. Moreover, your body doesn't shift abruptly from one energy source to another — the transition from one energetic pathway to another is very subtle. In a sense, all three metabolic processes overlap each other. So, if you can improve the effi-ciency of your energy systems through cross training then you can also improve your performance potential.

To summarize: The predominant energetic system used during activities that require 30 seconds or less is your ATP-PC System. Activities requiring be-tween 30 - 90 seconds use a blend of your ATP-PC System and Anaerobic Glycolysis. For activities that are between 1.5 - 3.0 minutes in duration, energy is provided by the collective efforts of Anaerobic Glycolysis and your Aerobic System. After three minutes of continuous activity, your Aerobic System predominates.

THE "ULTIMATE PUMP"

The most important muscle in your body is your heart — a large, hollow muscle that is located just behind your sternum (or breastbone). Your heart is the primary driving force behind your three energy systems. The human heart is a cone-shaped organ about 5 inches long, 3.5 inches wide and 2.5 inches thick — roughly the size of a man's clenched fist. The average adult male heart weighs about 10 ounces while its female counterpart weighs about 8 ounces.

Your heart is the ultimate endurance muscle or "pump" — it contracts about 100,000 times each day, pausing only briefly after a contraction to fill with more blood for its next contraction. This muscular pump is comprised of left and right halves. Each half of your heart consists of two chambers: an atrium and a ventricle. The atria are the recovery chambers of your heart and the ventricles are the pumping chambers.

Your blood has two routes or circuits: the Systemic Circuit and the Pulmonary Circuit. In the Systemic Circuit, the powerful left ventricle of your heart pumps oxygen-enriched blood to your body tissues (such as your skeletal muscles). The blood collects carbon dioxide and other metabolic wastes and returns to the right atrium of your heart. In the Pulmonary Circuit, the right ventricle of your heart sends oxygen-deficient blood that is laden with carbon dioxide to your lungs. The blood drops off carbon dioxide, picks up oxygenated blood and returns to the left atrium of your heart.

Normally, the right half of your heart pumps the same amount of blood as the left half of the heart. However, the left half of your heart is much stronger and better developed than your right half. The reason for this is because the left half of your heart must pump blood throughout your entire body while the right half only has to pump blood to your lungs.

Your Blood Pressure

When your heart forces blood through your blood vessels, the fluid is under pressure. Your blood pressure is a measure of the force exerted by your blood against the arterial walls. Blood pressure actually has two measures: systolic

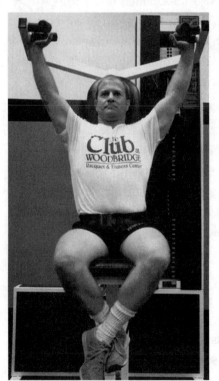

and diastolic. Your systolic blood pressure is the maximum pressure in your arteries during ventricular contraction; your diastolic blood pressure is the maximum pressure during ventricular relaxation — that is, when your heart relaxes between beats as the atria and ventricles fill with blood.

Blood pressure is measured in millimeters of mercury (mmHg). In males, a normal resting blood pressure is about 120/70 mmHg with the upper number being the systolic pressure and the lower number the diastolic pressure; in females, a normal resting blood pressure is about 8 - 10 mmHg lower. High blood pressure — or

Left: Active individuals usually have lower resting heart rates than sedentary individuals. (photo by Matt Brzycki)

hypertension — is when the resting blood pressures exceed 140/90 mmHg. (Those with chronic hypertension should seek medical consultation.)

Exercise influences your systolic blood pressure more than your diastolic. Your systolic blood pressure increases in proportion to your exercise intensity and can rise to 200 mmHg or more. During intense activity, the diastolic blood pressure of healthy individuals remains the same or drops slightly. (An increase in diastolic blood pressure during exercise is considered abnormal and cause for alarm.) Maximum blood pressure usually occurs at maximum heart rate.

Your Heart Rate

As the blood surges out of the ventricles, it pounds the arterial wall. This impact is transmitted along the length of the artery and can be felt as a throb or a "pulse" at those points where an artery lies just under your skin. The beat of your pulse is synchronous with the beat of your heart. To a degree, the rate of the heartbeat is dependent upon the size of the organism. In general, the smaller the size the faster the heartbeat. A normal resting heart rate for humans is about 60 - 80 beats per minute (bpm). Women's hearts beat 6 - 8 times per minute faster than those of men. Children's hearts beat even more rapidly — as high as 130 bpm at birth. Animals larger than humans have slower heart rates — an elephant has one of only 20 bpm. On the other hand, a shrew's heart beats 1,000 times per minute.

Active individuals usually have lower resting heart rates than sedentary individuals; in fact, some highly fit people have resting heart rates of less than 40 bpm. A lower resting heart rate may be especially important if the heart is limited to a certain number of beats over the course of a lifetime. For instance, suppose that the human heart is confined to about 2.5 billion beats before it simply wears out from the labors of continual usage. In this scenario, a person with an average resting heart rate of 70 bpm could expect to live a little less than 68 years; on the other hand, someone with an average resting heart rate of 60 bpm could expect to live a little more than 79 years. If this concept were true, a decrease in the resting heart rate of just 10 bpm would translate into more than 11 additional years of life. While this notion is intriguing, it has yet to have been proven scientifically. Nevertheless, it does generate the possibility of added importance in having a lower resting heart rate.

The Training Effect

Like all muscle tissue, exercise causes your heart to get larger or "hypertrophy." (Its inverse — a decrease in muscular size — is known as "atrophy.")

Specifically, its ventricular wall becomes thicker from anaerobic exercise (e.g., activities of high intensity and short duration such as strength training) and its ventricular cavity becomes larger from aerobic exercise (e.g., activities of low intensity and long duration such as long-distance running). This adaptation permits your heart to accept more blood and to expel it more powerfully. As your heart becomes a better conditioned muscle, its ability to circulate blood also improves.

Your stroke volume is the amount of blood pumped by your heart per beat. If you are a male, each beat of your heart may pump anywhere from .07 - .12 liters of blood while you are at rest. During intense exercise, stroke volume may increase to 0.2 liters of blood per beat or more. In general, females have lower values for stroke volume than males under all conditions — which is probably due to the fact that the size of the female heart is, on average, smaller than that of her male counterpart. Finally, someone with a high level of fitness has a greater stroke volume than someone with a low level of fitness.

Cardiac output is the amount of blood pumped by your heart per minute. It is the product of your stroke volume and your heart rate. At rest, the volume of blood pumped by your heart is about 5 liters per minute (L/min). During vigorous exercise, the amount of blood pumped may increase to more than 25 L/min. Females tend to have a slightly higher cardiac output than males when exercising at the same level of intensity.

When exercising, your stroke volume increases progressively up to a certain point and then it levels off. In other words, there's a physiological limit to the amount of blood that your heart can pump. Once your stroke volume is maximal, further increases in your cardiac output are possible only through increases in your heart rate. As your level of fitness improves, the point at which your stroke volume reaches a steady-state value becomes higher.

Once again, your resting heart rate is lowered as a direct result of exercise — especially from aerobic activities. A slower heart rate coupled with a larger stroke volume — that is, the ejection of a larger volume of blood — indicates an efficient circulatory system. This is true because your heart won't beat as often for a given cardiac output. If your heart pumps more blood per beat and needs less beats to function, you've increased the proficiency of your muscular pump. As an example, if your resting heart rate is 71 bpm and your heart ejects .07 liters of blood per beat then your resting cardiac output is about 5 L/min [71 bpm x .07 liters per beat = 4.97 L/min].

As a result of improved fitness, let's say that you've increased your stroke volume to .08 liters of blood per beat. In this case, you would need a resting heart rate of only 62 bpm in order to produce the same resting cardiac output of roughly 5 L/min [62 bpm x .08 liters per beat = 4.96 L/min]. So, for the same resting cardiac output your heart would pump a greater volume of blood using less beats — a characteristic of an efficient circulatory system.

THE RESPIRATORY PROCESS

Respiration is a combination of inspiration and expiration. Inspiration — or inhalation — is an active process in which your lungs inflate and air enters your body. The primary muscle of respiration is your diaphragm — a large, dome-shaped sheet of muscle located in your upper abdominal cavity. Expiration — or exhalation — is a passive process in which your lungs deflate and air is released into the environment. During vigorous exercise, however, expiration is an active process that is facilitated by your abdominal muscles and your internal intercostal muscles (which lie between your ribs along with your external intercostal muscles).

The respiratory process is accomplished without continuous conscious effort. Actually, respiration is a rhythmic action: Inflation of your lungs during inspiration causes expiration; deflation of your lungs during expiration causes inspiration.

At rest, a healthy adult's respiration rate is about 10 - 12 breaths per minute. During strenuous exercise, your frequency of respiration may increase to 40 - 50 breaths per minute. The volume of air entering or leaving your lungs during a single breath is known as your "tidal volume." Under resting conditions, your tidal volume is around 0.5 liters of oxygen per breath and may increase to about 3.0 liters of oxygen per breath during intense activity.

Your respiratory system has two major functions: to exchange gases (i.e., to deliver oxygen and to eliminate carbon dioxide) and to maintain your acid-base balance.

The Gas Exchange

Your diaphragm — with assistance from your external intercostal muscles in conjunction with the natural changes of pressures within your body — produces an open trade of oxygen and carbon dioxide. The venous blood sent to your lungs by the right ventricle is low in oxygen and high in carbon dioxide. In the lungs, your blood unloads carbon dioxide and loads oxygen. The blood returns to the left atrium as arterial blood that is high in oxygen and low in carbon dioxide.

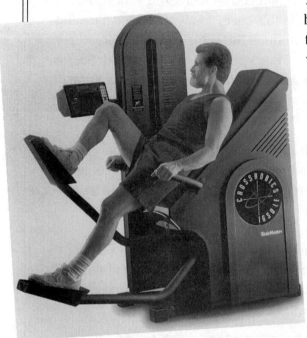

A second exchange of gases occurs between your blood and tissues. In this case, your thickly-muscled left ventricle pumps arterial blood to your tissues. Once again, the blood delivers oxygen and removes carbon dioxide. Essentially, this trade of gases converts arterial blood to venous blood. The venous blood returns to your right atrium where the entire process of gas exchange and transport is repeated over and over again.

Acid-Base Balance

The respiratory process also regulates your acid-base balance — that is, the pH of your body. Recall that lactic acid is a direct end-product of anaerobic training and is the prime suspect in muscular fatigue. Without a system to remove or "buffer" this metabolite, your body fluids would become more acidic and unsettle your delicate acid-base balance.

Your pH is a direct measure of acidity or alkalinity. The lower the pH, the greater the acidity — a pH that is less than 7.0 is considered acidic while a pH that is greater than 7.0 is considered alkaline. (A pH of 7.0 is neutral.) During intense exercise, the increased production of carbon dioxide and lactic acid may briefly lower your muscle pH from a normal resting value of about 7.0 to a level of 6.4. (In human muscle, pH values as low as 6.25 have been recorded.) The lactate diffuses from your muscles into neighboring tissues and ultimately overflows into your blood. This causes your blood pH to temporarily drop from a normal resting level of about 7.4 to as low as 6.8. An environment that is too acidic may inhibit several chemical reactions that are needed for energy production or may result in pain, distress and muscle fatigue. So, your acid-base system is basically an alarm mechanism that alerts you to reduce your level of effort because your acid levels have become too high.

Above: It's critical that you make your cross-training activities progressively more challenging in order to provide an overload and produce further physiological improvements in the target system. (Photo provided by StairMaster Sports/ Medical Products, Inc.)

Unfortunately, blood lactate is always created during anaerobic activity. What separates individuals who are highly fit from those who are out-of-shape is the degree to which lactic acid can be tolerated and how quickly it can be metabolized. As you improve your fitness through cross training, you will be better suited to discard waste products, exchange gases and neutralize the metabolically-produced acids thereby delaying muscular fatigue. Otherwise, you must abbreviate — or perhaps even terminate — your activities until you attain a more acceptable metabolic environment.

PHYSIOLOGICAL OVERLOAD

Any type of cross-training activity — whether it be for aerobic, anaerobic, strength, flexibility or metabolic improvements — must incorporate a well-known foundational concept in exercise physiology called the "Overload Principle." "Overload" means that a particular physiological system must be made to work harder than it is accustomed to working. This suggests that there is a minimum threshold level that must be surpassed before a specific, long-term adaptation occurs.

Over a period of time, you'll likely find that the same cross-training workout — which was originally difficult — can be performed with less exertion. As such, it's critical that you make your cross-training activities progressively more challenging in order to provide an overload and produce further physiological improvements in the target system (i.e., your musculoskeletal, circulatory and/or respiratory system).

Because of this, it's important for you to keep accurate records of your cross-training performances. Maintaining records of your key program components allows you to keep track of your progress thereby making your workouts more productive and more meaningful.

GENETIC INFLUENCES

The most important factor that influences your anaerobic and aerobic potential is your inherited characteristics or your genetics. For the most part, you cannot change the qualities that you've acquired from your ancestors. Stated otherwise, you have no control over what you've inherited.

The "genetic profile" of someone who has a high level of aerobic ability differs greatly from that of someone who has a high level of anaerobic ability. One of the most influential of all inherited traits in your genetic portfolio is your predominant muscle-fiber type. Your muscle fibers may be grouped into two major categories: fast twitch (FT) and slow twitch (ST). These two major fiber types differ in several areas including speed of contraction, force of contraction and endurance capacity. Your FT fibers can contract quickly and generate large amounts of force, but they fatigue rather easily. Relative to FT muscle fibers, your ST fibers contract slower and produce less force but they have greater endurance. Because of their fatigue characteristics, FT fibers are often referred to as being glycolytic and ST fibers as oxidative. (Some researchers also recognize one or more interme-diate fiber types that possess characteristics of both FT and ST fibers.)

 Your muscles are composed of both fiber types and the different types are intermingled throughout each muscle. However, the actual percentage and distribution pattern of your FT and ST fibers is genetically determined — it is established by the time you are born and remains relatively constant for the remainder of your life. Some individuals have inherited a predominant fiber type that increases their performance potential in certain activities. For example, an accomplished sprinter is capable of generating tremendous amounts of force in a rather short period of time. A high percentage of FT fibers would be revealed by a microscopic analysis of a muscle-tissue sample taken from a sprinter's lower-body musculature. The same holds true for any other person whose success is predicated upon quick, powerful movements. On the other hand, a successful long-distance runner has a high capacity for endurance. A high distribution of ST fibers would be dis-closed by a microscopic analysis of a muscle-tissue sample taken from the lower body of a distance runner or any other individual who excels in pro-longed, endurance-type activities. It should also be noted that your fiber-type mixture may differ from one muscle to another and may even vary from one side of your body to the other.

Except for identical twins, each person is a unique genetic entity with a different genetic potential. Some people are predisposed toward being more proficient at aerobic activities while others are destined to become more successful at anaerobic activities. Regardless of your genetic destiny, your goal should be to realize your physical potential by cross training for fitness.

4
Aerobic Cross Training

The most important aspect of your physical profile and the best indicator of your overall health is your aerobic fitness. Specifically, your aerobic fitness is a measure of how well your muscles consume, transport and utilize oxygen during physical exertions. The best way for you to improve these physiological mechanisms is through aerobic cross training.

The metabolic pathway that is responsible for your aerobic fitness is your Aerobic System (which is important in efforts that are of prolonged duration.) Therefore, the primary target of your aerobic cross training is your Aerobic System.

From a competitive standpoint, an athlete who has a high level of aerobic fitness surrenders to fatigue less quickly than an opponent who has a low level of aerobic fitness — regardless of the sport or activity. Besides this physiological adaptation, aerobic cross training — when used in conjunction with proper dieting — helps maintain your percentage of body fat at an acceptable level.

When cross training for fitness, it's critical to first establish a solid foundation of aerobic support. The more finely-tuned your Aerobic System becomes, the better your anaerobic systems are able to function. In order to perform anaerobically, your Aerobic System must operate as efficiently and as effectively as possible to provide physiological support for your anaerobic systems.

The message is clear: By improving your aerobic fitness, your heart and all of your metabolic systems can function more productively and more efficiently.

AEROBIC GUIDELINES

Your aerobic fitness may be developed and maintained by using several easy-to-follow guidelines. These guidelines have been developed by the American College of Sports Medicine (ACSM) based upon the existing scientific evidence concerning exercise prescription for healthy adults and can be organized under the acronym FITT, which stands for Frequency, Intensity, Time and Type. (Most sedentary individuals can safely begin an exercise program of moderate intensity. However, the ACSM recommends that males at or above the age of 40 and females at or above the age of 50 receive a medical examination before beginning a vigorous exercise program.)

Frequency

In order to improve your aerobic fitness, the ACSM and many other exercise authorities suggest that you perform an appropriate aerobic activity 3 - 5 days per week. Exercising less than two days per week does not appear adequate enough to promote any meaningful changes in your aerobic capacity. The amount of improvement from training aerobically more than five days per week is negligible.

Doing aerobic activities more frequently is beneficial when weight reduction is a goal. However, beginning with too much exercise too soon may very well lead to an overuse injury such as tendinitis. This is especially true of certain populations including younger and physically immature teens, older adults and those who have been inactive or are in poor physical condition. Individuals who are susceptible to overuse injuries should perform an aerobic workout 2 - 3 days per week to reduce their potential for orthopedic problems. As these individuals adjust and adapt to the unfamiliar physical demands, their dosage of aerobic activity can be increased to 3 - 5 weekly workouts.

Intensity

Other than your genetics, the most important component of your aerobic cross training is your level of intensity or effort. Your heart rate increases in direct proportion to the intensity of the activity. As such, your exercising heart rate is commonly used as an estimate of your aerobic intensity. Since there is a slight but steady decrease in your maximal heart rate with aging, estimates of your maximal heart rate are made on the basis of your age. The

Right: An athlete who has a high level of aerobic fitness surrenders to fatigue less quickly than an opponent who has a low level of aerobic fitness. (Photo by Larry French)

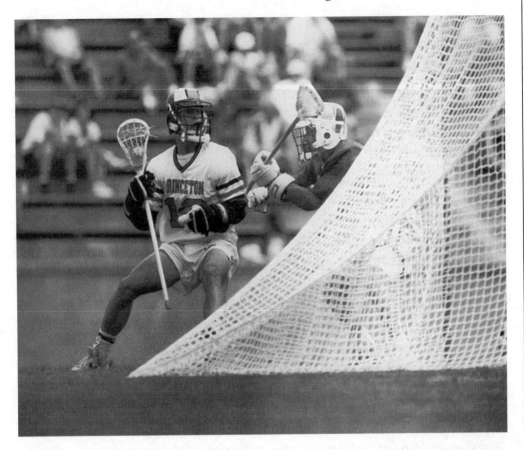

ACSM recommends that you maintain a level of 60 - 90 percent of your age-predicted maximum heart rate to receive an aerobic-training benefit. (Previously, the ACSM recommended exercising at 70 - 85 percent of the age-predicted maximum heart rate. In 1990, the ACSM expanded their guideline presumably to encompass extremes in the population — the poorly conditioned and the highly conditioned.)

To find a rough estimate of your age-predicted maximum heart rate in beats per minute (bpm), simply subtract your age from 220. For example, the age-predicted maximum heart rate of a 30-year-old individual is 190 bpm [220 - 30 = 190]. To find the recommended heart-rate training zone, multiply 190 bpm by .60 and .90. This means that a 30-year-old individual needs to maintain an exercise heart rate between about 114 - 171 bpm to elicit an aerobic conditioning effect [190 bpm x .60 = 114 bpm; 190 bpm x .90 = 171 bpm].

In the case of maximal heart rate, it's important to note that the equation "220 minus age" has a standard deviation of about 11 bpm. Considering all 30-year-old individuals, this means that about 68.26 percent of them have maximal heart rates between 179 - 201 bpm, 95.44 percent between 168 - 212 bpm and 99.73 percent between 157 - 223 bpm.

Some people may need to maintain their heart rates above their recommended training zone. For instance, if you are highly active or have an above-average level of fitness you must exercise at a greater percentage of your age-predicted maximum heart rate to receive a sufficient cardiac workload.

Because of potential health risks and possible compliance problems, it may be necessary for others to maintain their heart rates below their recommended training zone. If you are sedentary or have a relatively low level of fitness you should exercise at a lower percentage of your age-predicted maximum heart rate. Exercising at a lower intensity may also be necessary in the early stages of aerobic cross training.

Remember, a favorable response depends upon exercising with an appropriate level of intensity or effort. Intensity is a relative term that depends upon each individual's level of fitness. For some people, training with a lower percentage of their age-predicted maximum heart rate may actually represent a high level of intensity and an adequate cardiac workload for them. Stated otherwise, exercise of low intensity for an active individual may be of high intensity for a sedentary individual. Depending upon the initial level of fitness, exercising at an intensity below the suggested range can actually produce some improvement in aerobic fitness.

To determine an appropriate level of effort, you should adjust your intensity depending upon whether the activity (or exercise) feels too easy or too difficult. If it feels uncomfortable, reduce your intensity; if it feels easy, increase your intensity. Also keep in mind that your intensity (and your heart rate) is influenced by many factors including the environmental temperature, your body position and the muscles being exercised.

Your heart rate can be easily measured at several different sites on your body. Numerous heart-rate monitors are available commercially that can give you a reasonably accurate reading of your heart rate. However, the easiest and least expensive way to determine your heart rate is to measure it yourself. This can be done by locating your pulse at either the carotid artery (in your neck) or the radial artery (in your wrist). Simply place the tips of your index and middle fingers over one of these sites. (During intense exercise, your carotid and radial arteries are easy to find.) Immediately after a session of aerobic cross training, count your pulse for 10 seconds. Multiplying that number by 6 gives you a good estimate of your exercise heart rate for one minute. A similar estimate can also be obtained by counting your pulse for 15 seconds and multiplying that number by 4.

Time

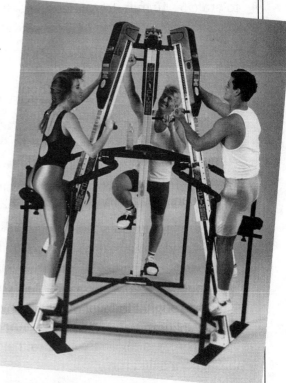

The ACSM recommends that you exercise continuously for a minimum of 20 minutes and a maximum of 60 minutes in order for you to receive a favorable aerobic-training benefit. The duration of the activity is inversely proportional to the intensity of the activity. So, the duration of your effort can be relatively brief provided that your level of intensity is high. As an example, a review of the literature by the ACSM suggests that exercising for a duration of as little as 10 - 15 minutes can significantly improve your aerobic ability. However, a workout this brief would have to be extremely intense in order to produce an aerobic-training effect. In general, investing 20 minutes of continuous activity with an appropriate level of intensity is adequate enough to improve your aerobic fitness.

It should also be noted that if the length of your aerobic effort is too brief, your workout might not produce a desirable caloric expenditure. This may be an important consideration — particularly if your primary objective is weight reduction. If losing weight is your main intention, you should perform aerobic-type activities for 30 - 60 minutes. (Additional guidelines for a safe weight-loss program are detailed in Chapter 9.)

When your intensity is low, your activities should be conducted for a longer period of time to induce an aerobic-training benefit. However, lengthy aerobic workouts may be inappropriate for some people in the initial stages of a fitness program. First of all, performing too much exercise too soon increases the risk of incurring an overuse injury. Secondly, some individuals may initially have such low levels of fitness that they may only be able to

Above: The best advice is for you to select activities that are enjoyable, compatible with your skill levels and orthopedically safe. (Photo provided by Heart Rate, Inc.)

tolerate 5 - 10 minutes of aerobic activity. In either case, the length of the aerobic sessions can be gradually increased as their fitness levels improve.

Type

If the frequency, intensity and duration of your aerobic cross-training workouts are similar (i.e., in terms of total caloric/energy expenditure), your physiological adaptations will be the same — regardless of the aerobic activity. Therefore, you can use a variety of cross-training activities to obtain an aerobic-conditioning effect.

The preferred types of aerobic activities are those that require a continuous effort, are rhythmic in nature and involve large amounts of muscle mass. Traditional outdoor aerobic activities that can be used to meet these criteria include cross-country skiing, cycling, hiking/backpacking, ice/in-line (or roller) skating, jogging/running, rowing and walking; popular indoor activities are aerobic dancing, rope jumping, swimming and stationary exercises on specialized equipment such as rowers, cycles (upright or recumbent), motorized treadmills and stair climbers/steppers. Most of these aerobic options are recreational activities that can be performed — and enjoyed — throughout a lifetime.

You can obtain aerobic benefits from activities such as soccer, basketball and racquet sports. However, your intensity level can vary a great deal during these activities due to their intermittent nature. The way these activities are structured also influences your level of intensity: Playing full-court is generally more demanding than half-court; playing a singles match is generally more demanding than a doubles match.

To avoid boredom, it's important for you to change activities from time to time. Fortunately, aerobic cross training permits a large amount of variety in terms of your exercise selections.

Each aerobic activity has its advantages and disadvantages. For instance, swimming is desirable because it's a non-weightbearing activity — the water supports your bodyweight which virtually eliminates the compressive forces on your bones, joints and connective tissue. On the other hand, swimming requires a certain degree of proficiency. If you have poor swimming skills, your exercising heart rate may exceed your recommended training zone in a struggle just to keep yourself afloat. If you aren't skilled at swimming, you'll also tire very quickly. Therefore, swimming isn't a good aerobic option for anyone with poor swimming fundamentals. However, swimming represents an excellent choice if your skills are adequate.

In addition, some activities aren't advisable if you are prone to injury or are likely to complicate an existing orthopedic condition. For instance, rope jumping is a high-impact, weightbearing activity that has a greater risk of orthopedic stress and overuse injuries than low-impact, non-weightbearing activities. As such, rope jumping isn't recommended if you are a larger-than-average person (larger due to either fat tissue or muscle tissue) because of the excessive stress on your ankles, knees and lower back. Likewise, a woman who jumps rope during pregnancy may endanger her fetus. Further-more, someone with chronic low-back pain would be more comfortable cycling in a recumbent position instead of in the traditional upright position due to the decreased amount of stress on the lumbar spine. So, the best advice is for you to select suitable activities that are enjoyable, compatible with your skill levels and orthopedically safe.

If you are an athlete preparing for a specific event — such as running or swimming — the best activities to do are the ones you're going to perform in competition. If you want to become a better runner, you must primarily run; if you want to become a better swimmer, you must primarily swim. Other-wise, the best activities are the ones you enjoy the most. As long as it's orthopedically appropriate, the equipment you choose to strengthen your heart isn't as critical as your intensity and the duration of the activity. Your heart doesn't know if you pedaled on a recumbent cycle one day and ran on a motorized treadmill the next. The only thing that really matters is whether or not you applied a meaningful workload to your heart and Aerobic System. (Cross-training options are detailed in Chapter 10.)

APPROPRIATE AEROBIC EXERCISE

In a nutshell, you should perform aerobic cross training at a frequency, intensity and duration that is developmentally appropriate and orthopedi-cally safe while using suitable activities that require a sustained effort. If you are a healthy adult, your specific exercise prescription is to perform aerobic activities 3 - 5 times per week [frequency] at 60 - 90 percent of your age-predicted maximum heart rate [intensity] for 20 - 60 consecutive minutes [time] using appropriate activities that require a prolonged effort [type]. Remember, all of these guidelines must be included in your aerobic cross training in order to improve your fitness.

MEANINGFUL AEROBIC EXERCISE

Over a period of time, you'll likely find that the same aerobic workout — which was originally difficult — can be performed with less exertion. As you become more fit, your exercising heart rate will be lower for a given level of intensity. Because of this, you must increase your intensity as needed so that you are always exercising at an appropriate percentage of your maximum heart rate. In addition, your ability to maintain a higher training heart rate becomes easier. As such, it's important to understand that your aerobic cross-training activities need to be progressively more challenging in order for you to make further improvements in your aerobic fitness.

To ensure that you produce continued aerobic improvements, you can progressively overload your Aerobic System by (1) completing the same distance at a faster pace (i.e., in a shorter amount of time); (2) covering a greater distance at the same pace; or (3) gradually increasing both the distance and the pace. As an example, suppose you cycled 4 miles in 20 minutes. In a future aerobic workout, you should try to either cycle 4 miles in less than 20 minutes, cycle more than 4 miles in 20 minutes or cycle slightly more than 4 miles in a little less than 20 minutes. Either way, you made your Aerobic System work harder than it was accustomed to working.

Consequently, it's important for you to keep accurate records of your aerobic cross-training performances. Maintaining records allows you to keep track of your progress thereby making your workouts more productive and more meaningful. During aerobic cross-training, the key program components to monitor include the duration of your workouts, the distances you complete, the frequency of your training and your intensity levels (i.e., your exercise heart rate).

PREDICTING OXYGEN INTAKE

Oxygen intake — or oxygen consumption — is a very reliable and widely-accepted indicator of your level of aerobic fitness. Like virtually all of your other physiological characteristics, your aerobic potential is greatly influenced by your genetics. Your oxygen intake is also affected by your age, gender and body size.

There are a number of ways to accurately measure oxygen intake in a laboratory. One way is to step up to and down from a bench of a standard height at a fixed rate of stepping. Another way is to pedal a cycle ergometer (i.e., a device that measures work) in an upright or a recumbent position using your legs and/or arms. In terms of assessing oxygen intake, the most widely-used laboratory apparatus is probably the motor-driven treadmill. Each of these devices makes it possible for you to exercise at different levels of intensity while maintaining your body in a relatively stable position. This allows you to be instrumented in order to measure your various physiological responses. For example, your expired air can be collected and analyzed to determine the exact amount of oxygen being consumed as well as the response of your heart rate, blood pressure and body temperature.

Laboratory testing is an excellent means of providing you with accurate and valid data. For the average person, however, laboratory testing can be expensive, time-consuming and impractical. Fortunately, there is a much more practical way of assessing your oxygen intake without having the drawbacks of laboratory testing. Since these assessments are performed outside the laboratory, they are referred to as "field tests." Certain field tests have a high correlation to laboratory tests of oxygen consumption. One of the most popular field tests used to determine oxygen intake is the 1.5-Mile Running Test. (A 1-Mile Running Test is more suitable for adolescents and the elderly.) The primary objective of this test is to run 1.5 miles in the least amount of time. For this field test to be as accurate as possible, you must run exactly 1.5 miles and it must be on a level surface. Because of this, running on an indoor or outdoor track is preferred. Generally, the results of the 1.5-Mile Running Test are an excellent predictor of your oxygen intake. However, it's important to realize that this test of aerobic fitness favors runners since it involves running.

Table 4.1 lists predicted values of oxygen intake based upon the time you take to complete a 1.5-mile run. Various running times are given in 5-second intervals between 8:00 - 15:55. These values are an absolute measure of how much oxygen you consumed in milliliters per kilogram of your bodyweight per minute (or ml/kg/min). Table 4.2 shows norms for oxygen consumption in absolute terms based upon your age and gender.

Oxygen Consumption: Absolute

Let's suppose that a 30-year-old man weighs 198 pounds and can run 1.5 miles in 12:30. Note in Table 4.1 that his oxygen intake for this particular running time is 42.12 ml/kg/min — or simply 42.12. In other words, he consumed about 42.12 milliliters of oxygen for every kilogram that he weighed during each minute of his 1.5-mile run. Referring to Table 4.2 (under 30 - 39-year-old males), note that this value [42.12] falls between the range of 40 - 47. This indicates that his level of aerobic fitness would be considered average. (Elite male endurance athletes — such as cross-country runners and skiers — have recorded oxygen intake values as high as the upper 70s to low 80s.)

Time	Value	Time	Value	Time	Value	Time	Value
8:00	63.84	10:00	51.77	12:00	43.73	14:00	37.98
8:05	63.22	10:05	51.37	12:05	43.45	14:05	37.77
8:10	62.61	10:10	50.98	12:10	43.17	14:10	37.57
8:15	62.01	10:15	50.59	12:15	42.90	14:15	37.37
8:20	61.42	10:20	50.21	12:20	42.64	14:20	37.18
8:25	60.85	10:25	49.84	12:25	42.38	14:25	36.98
8:30	60.29	10:30	49.47	12:30	42.12	14:30	36.79
8:35	59.74	10:35	49.11	12:35	41.86	14:35	36.60
8:40	59.20	10:40	48.75	12:40	41.61	14:40	36.41
8:45	58.67	10:45	48.40	12:45	41.36	14:45	36.23
8:50	58.15	10:50	48.06	12:50	41.11	14:50	36.04
8:55	57.63	10:55	47.72	12:55	40.87	14:55	35.86
9:00	57.13	11:00	47.38	13:00	40.63	15:00	35.68
9:05	56.64	11:05	47.05	13:05	40.39	15:05	35.50
9:10	56.16	11:10	46.73	13:10	40.16	15:10	35.33
9:15	55.68	11:15	46.41	13:15	39.93	15:15	35.15
9:20	55.21	11:20	46.09	13:20	39.70	15:20	34.98
9:25	54.76	11:25	45.78	13:25	39.48	15:25	34.81
9:30	54.31	11:30	45.47	13:30	39.26	15:30	34.64
9:35	53.87	11:35	45.17	13:35	39.04	15:35	34.48
9:40	53.43	11:40	44.87	13:40	38.82	15:40	34.31
9:45	53.01	11:45	44.58	13:45	38.61	15:45	34.15
9:50	52.59	11:50	44.29	13:50	38.39	15:50	33.99
9:55	52.18	11:55	44.01	13:55	38.19	15:55	33.83

Table 4.1: Predicted Values of Oxygen Uptake Based Upon the Time to Complete a 1.5-mile Run

Table 4.1 is only valid for determining your oxygen intake during a 1.5-mile run. The ACSM offers this formula for determining oxygen intake in ml/kg/min for a run of any known distance and duration:

oxygen intake = (speed in m/min) x (0.2 ml/kg/min per m/min) + 3.5 ml/kg/min

As an example, imagine that a woman just completed a 5,000-meter race in 20:00. In this case, her running speed was 250 meters per minute [5,000 meters divided by 20 minutes]. Next, multiply her speed [250 m/min] by the oxygen cost of horizontal running [0.2 ml/kg/min per m/min] and add the oxygen cost at rest [3.5 ml/kg/min]. This calculation yields a value of 53.5 ml/kg/min [250 m/min x .2 ml/kg/min per m/min + 3.5 ml/kg/min = 53.5 ml/kg/min]. For this formula to be accurate, you must run on a level surface at a speed of at least 5 miles per hour (mph) or 134 m/min. (To convert mph to m/min, multiply the mph by 26.8; to convert miles to meters, multiply the number of miles by 1,609.)

A similar formula can be used to determine oxygen intake for walking speeds between 1.9 - 3.7 mph. At lower speeds, walking is generally a more efficient process than running. In fact, the oxygen cost of horizontal walking at a given speed is about one half that for running. Therefore, the only difference in the previously mentioned formula is that the walking speed is multiplied by 0.1 ml/kg/min per m/min (the oxygen cost of horizontal walking) and then added to 3.5 ml/kg/min (the oxygen cost at rest). So, if you walked 2,700 meters in 30 minutes, your oxygen intake would be 12.5 ml/kg/min [90 m/min x .1 ml/kg/min per m/min + 3.5 ml/kg/min = 12.5 ml/kg/min].

Oxygen Consumption: Relative

Oxygen intake can also be expressed in relative terms in liters per minute (L/min). Determining oxygen intake in relative terms is usually a better indicator of your aerobic fitness because the value takes into account differences in bodyweight. For instance, if two people ran the same distance in the same time, they would consume the same amount of oxygen per unit of bodyweight in absolute terms. In relative terms, however, a larger individual would actually consume more oxygen than a smaller individual because a greater body mass was displaced over a given distance.

To determine your oxygen intake in L/min, you must first convert your bodyweight to kilograms (kg). To do this, divide your bodyweight in pounds (lb) by 2.2. Using the earlier example of the 30-year-old male, his 198-pound bodyweight is equal to 90 kg [198 lb divided by 2.2 kg/lb = 90 kg]. Next, multiply his bodyweight (in kilograms) by his oxygen intake (in ml/kg/min) and divide by 1,000 (to convert from milliliters to liters). Staying with the same example as before, his bodyweight [90 kg] multiplied by his oxygen intake [42.12 ml/kg/min] is 3,790.8 ml/min. To divide by 1,000, simply move

Women					
Age	**Low**	**Fair**	**Average**	**Good**	**High**
20-29	<28	29-34	35-43	44-48	49+
30-39	<27	28-33	34-41	42-47	48+
40-49	<25	26-31	32-40	41-45	46+
50-59	<21	22-28	29-36	37-41	42+
60-69	<17	18-22	23-31	32-36	37+

Men					
Age	**Low**	**Fair**	**Average**	**Good**	**High**
20-29	<38	39-43	44-51	52-56	57+
30-39	<34	35-39	40-47	48-51	52+
40-49	<30	31-35	36-43	44-47	48+
50-59	<25	26-31	32-39	40-43	44+
60-69	<21	22-26	27-35	36-39	40+

Table 4.2: Norms for Oxygen Intake in Absolute Terms (From Astrand 1960; Vanderburgh and Considine 1995)

the decimal point three places to the left. This means that a 198-pound individual who ran 1.5 miles in 12:30 would consume about 3.79 liters of oxygen during every minute of his run.

Table 4.3 lists norms for oxygen consumption in relative terms based upon your age, gender and bodyweight. Referring to this table (again under 30 - 39-year-old males), you'll find that this value [3.79 L/min] is considered to be an excellent level of fitness for males of his age relative to his bodyweight. Recall that when his bodyweight wasn't considered, his level of aerobic fitness was considered average. As such, oxygen intake is a more accurate indicator of your fitness level when it is expressed relative to your bodyweight in L/min. (Values of more than 5 - 6 L/min are fairly common in highly fit individuals.)

Oxygen-Consumption Expectations

According to the ACSM, the following regression equations can be used to predict your expected oxygen intake based upon your activity level, age and gender:

Active men: 69.7 – (.612 x age)
Active women: 42.9 – (.312 x age)
Sedentary men: 57.8 – (.445 x age)
Sedentary women: 42.3 – (.356 x age)

For instance, a sedentary 40-year-old woman would be expected to have an oxygen intake of about 28.06 ml/kg/min [42.3 minus the value of .356 x 40]. Comparing your expected oxygen intake to your actual oxygen intake is helpful in determining whether you have any Functional Aerobic Impairment (FAI). Your FAI may be found by subtracting your actual oxygen intake from your expected oxygen intake. This value is divided by your expected oxygen intake and then multiplied by 100 (to convert to a percentage). If the 40-year-old woman in this example was found to have an actual oxygen intake of 22.45 ml/kg/min, she would have an FAI of about 20 percent [her expected oxygen intake of 28.06 ml/kg/min minus her actual oxygen intake of 22.45 ml/kg/min divided by her expected oxygen intake of 28.06 ml/kg/min times 100 equals 19.99 percent]. A negative percentage indicates that your actual oxygen intake is better than expected. Once again, it must be noted that heredity plays an important role in determining your level of aerobic fitness.

Finally, the purpose of assessing your aerobic fitness should not be to compare your performance to that of another. It's unfair to make comparisons between people because everyone has a different genetic potential for

Women					
Age	Low	Fair	Average	Good	High
20-29	<1.69	1.70-1.99	2.00-2.49	2.50-2.79	2.80+
30-39	<1.59	1.60-1.89	1.90-2.39	2.40-2.69	2.70+
40-49	<1.49	1.50-1.79	1.80-2.29	2.30-2.59	2.60+
50-59	<1.39	1.40-1.69	1.70-2.19	2.20-2.49	2.50+
60-69	<1.29	1.30-1.59	1.60-2.09	2.10-2.39	2.40+

Men					
Age	Low	Fair	Average	Good	High
20-29	<2.79	2.80-3.09	3.10-3.69	3.70-3.99	4.00+
30-39	<2.49	2.50-2.79	2.80-3.39	3.40-3.69	3.70+
40-49	<2.19	2.20-2.49	2.50-3.09	3.10-3.39	3.40+
50-59	<1.89	1.90-2.19	2.20-2.79	2.80-3.09	3.10+
60-69	<1.59	1.60-1.89	1.90-2.49	2.50-2.79	2.80+

Table 4.3: Norms for Oxygen Intake in Relative Terms (From Astand 1960; Vanderburgh and Considine 1995)

achieving aerobic fitness. Fitness assessments are more meaningful and fair when your performance is compared to your last performance — not to the performance of others.

ESTIMATING CALORIC EXPENDITURE

A calorie is basically a unit of energy. In scientific terms, a calorie is defined as the amount of heat required to raise the temperature of one gram of water by one degree Celsius. In practical terms, a calorie is a measure of your energy intake (i.e., eating) and your energy expenditure (i.e., exercising).

The caloric equivalent of one liter of oxygen ranges from 4.7 calories when fats are used as the sole source of energy to 5.0 calories when carbohydrates are used as the only energy source. (The caloric equivalent of one liter of oxygen is 4.4 calories when proteins are used as the single source of energy. Under most circumstances, however, protein utilization during exercise is negligible in terms of energy production and is usually disregarded.) For all practical purposes — with little loss in precision — you use about 5 calories for every liter of oxygen that you consume. To determine your rate of caloric expenditure, simply take your oxygen intake value in L/min and multiply it by 5 calories per liter (cal/L). Recall the earlier example of the 198-pound male whose oxygen intake was 3.79 L/min. In this case, his rate of caloric expenditure would be almost 19 calories per minute [3.79 L/min x 5 cal/L = 18.95 cal/min].

To determine the total number of calories that were used during his 1.5-mile run, multiply his rate of caloric expenditure (in cal/min) by his running time.

In this case, multiplying 18.95 cal/min by 12.5 minutes (12:30 in decimal form) indicates that he used about 237 calories during his run [18.95 cal/min x 12.5 min = 237 cal].

MET LEVELS

Another way to quantify oxygen intake (and caloric/energy expenditure) is by assigning an activity a MET or Metabolic Equivalent. A MET is a multiple of your resting oxygen intake. One MET is defined as the amount of oxygen you consume while you are resting in a seated position — which is about 3.5 ml/kg/min. A level of 2 METs is equal to an oxygen intake of 7 ml/kg/min [3.5 ml/kg/min x 2 = 7 ml/kg/min]. Therefore, an activity that has a value of 2 METs requires twice as much oxygen (or energy) as complete rest (i.e., 7 ml/kg/min compared to 3.5 ml/kg/min); an activity that has a value of 6 METs requires three times as much oxygen as an activity that requires 2 METs (21 ml/kg/min compared to 7 ml/kg/min).

You can easily express your oxygen intake in METs. To do so, simply divide your oxygen intake in ml/kg/min by 3.5 ml/kg/min. For instance, the 198-pound male in the ongoing example had an oxygen intake of 42.12 ml/kg/min when he ran 1.5 miles in 12:30. In this case, his oxygen intake is equal to about 12 METs [42.12 divided by 3.5 ml/kg/min equals 12.03 METs].

You can also estimate your rate of caloric expenditure in calories per kilogram of your bodyweight per minute (cal/kg/min) and your calories per minute (cal/min) from your MET level. One MET is equal to about .0175 cal/kg/min. Therefore, your caloric expenditure can be estimated in cal/kg/min by multiplying your MET level by .0175 cal/kg/min. For example, the 198-pound male who recorded a MET level of 12.03 used about .210525 cal/min/kg [12.03 x .0175 cal/kg/min = .210525 cal/kg/min]. To estimate his cal/min, multiply his bodyweight in kilograms [90] by his cal/kg/min [.210525]. This yields a value of about 18.947 cal/min. (Note that his rate of caloric expenditure was previously estimated as 18.95 cal/min using a different series of calculations.)

Table 4.4 lists a wide range of cross-training activities along with estimates of cal/kg/min and MET levels which you can use to estimate your caloric expenditure. Remember, these are only estimates. Caloric expenditure during activities other than walking and running are difficult to predict. Your exact caloric expenditure depends heavily upon your skill at performing the activity and motivation. It is also influenced by the environmental conditions such as the wind, terrain, heat, humidity, altitude and air pollution. Nevertheless, this information still provides a reasonably accurate estimate of your caloric expenditure while cross training for fitness.

ACTIVITY	cal/kg/min	MET
aerobic dancing	.105	6.00
badminton, competitive	.147	8.40
badminton, recreational	.076	4.34
basketball, half-court	.088	5.03
basketball, full-court	.132	7.54
cycling, outdoor (10 mph)	.123	7.03
cycling (ergometer) 300 kpm	.065	3.71
600 kpm	.105	6.00
900 kpm	.149	8.51
1200 kpm	.193	11.03
dancing, ballroom		
rumba	.103	5.89
waltz	.084	4.80
golf	.085	4.86
handball	.143	8.17
hiking, 3 mph with a 40-pound pack	.100	5.71
judo	.195	11.14
karate	.195	11.14
mountain climbing	.147	8.40
racquetball	.143	8.17
rope jumping		
60 - 80 skips/min	.158	9.03
120 - 140 skips/min	.193	11.03
rowing, indoor (Concept II)		
2:32/500m (7.36 mph)	.118	6.74
2:16/500m (8.23 mph)	.140	8.00
2:00/500m (9.32 mph)	.175	10.00
running, level surface		
9 min/mi (6.67 mph)	.196	11.20
8 min/mi (7.50 mph)	.219	12.49
7 min/mi (8.57 mph)	.247	14.13
6 min/mi (10.0 mph)	.286	16.32
skating, recreational	.083	4.74
skiing, cross-country		
3 mph	.132	7.54
10 mph	.293	16.74
soccer	.132	7.54
squash	.143	8.17
stair climbing (StairMaster 4000PT)		
level 5	.114	6.51
level 9	.170	9.71
swimming, back stroke		
25 yd/min	.088	5.03
50 yd/min	.183	10.46
swimming, breast stroke		
25 yd/min	.088	5.03
50 yd/min	.183	10.46
swimming, front crawl		
25 yd/min	.088	5.03
50 yd/min	.183	10.46
swimming, side stroke (40 yd/min)	.161	9.20
tennis, competitive	.161	9.20
tennis, recreational	.103	5.89
volleyball, competitive	.117	6.69
volleyball, recreational	.051	2.91
walking, level asphalt road		
2.5 mph	.051	2.91
3.5 mph	.064	3.66
weight training	.116	6.63
weight training, circuit	.185	10.57

Table 4.4: Estimates of Caloric Expenditure (in cal/kg/min) and MET Levels for Selected Cross-training Activities

5 Anaerobic Cross Training

Many sports and activities are composed of brief, powerful movements that rely heavily upon your anaerobic abilities. The best way to prepare yourself for these specific physiological demands is anaerobic cross training.

The most common method of anaerobic cross training is to perform a series of all-out efforts of short duration such as sprinting. In order for your anaerobic activities to be most effective, they must be done in an organized manner. Performing anaerobic activities informally can be quite beneficial but a formal program that is structured and has a scientific basis is more precise and more productive.

Your anaerobic efforts must also be done in an aggressive and enthusiastic fashion. In addition, it's important to understand that manipulating the duration and the intensity of your efforts utilizes different anaerobic energy sources. A progressive system of short-term, high-intensity activities that are increasingly more challenging places a systematic overload on your anaerobic energy sources which helps you to realize your performance potential.

Finally, it should be noted that before you begin your anaerobic cross training, you must first establish a firm base of aerobic support. Your anaerobic systems cannot function at optimal levels without assistance from your Aerobic System. (Chapter 4 describes your Aerobic System in great detail.)

ANAEROBIC GUIDELINES

Anaerobic cross training is somewhat more complex than aerobic cross training. Your anaerobic systems play a significant role in activities that last anywhere from a split second to roughly three minutes — assuming, of

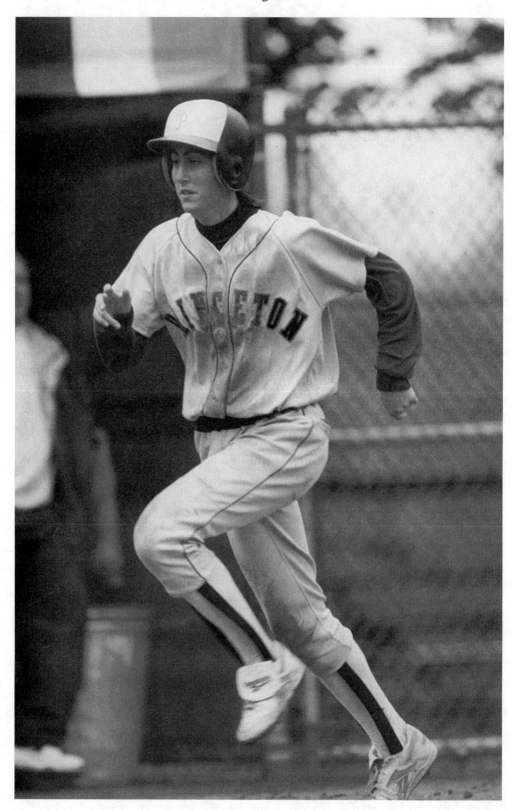

course, that your intensity of effort is great enough to elicit an anaerobic response. The complications arise because you have two energy sources — your ATP-PC System and Anaerobic Glycolysis — that operate within this anaerobic time span. Specifically, your ATP-PC System predominates during activities that are 30 seconds or less; activities that last between 30 - 90 seconds involve your ATP-PC System and Anaerobic Glycolysis; finally, Anaerobic Glycolysis — with an important helping hand from your Aerobic System — provides energy during activities that are between 1.5 - 3.0 minutes. (Your Aerobic System becomes your principal source of energy after about three minutes of continuous activity.)

Anaerobic intensity can be measured the same way as aerobic intensity: by monitoring your exercise heart rate. However, anaerobic cross training requires higher levels of intensity than aerobic cross training. In order to involve your anaerobic pathways, you must raise your heart rate to near-maximal levels for brief periods of time. Elevating your heart rate to more than 90 percent of your age-predicted maximum is usually a good indicator that you're utilizing your anaerobic pathways. (Chapter 4 describes how you can determine your age-predicted maximum heart rate.) At such high levels of intensity, you won't be able to exercise continuously for much more than about three minutes at a time.

If you are highly active or have an above-average level of fitness you must exercise at a greater percentage of your age-predicted maximum heart rate; if you are sedentary or have a relatively low level of fitness you should exercise at a lower percentage of your age-predicted maximum heart rate.

Remember, anaerobic cross training is characterized by high-intensity efforts performed over relatively brief periods of time. Unlike aerobic cross training — where a decreased level of intensity can be sacrificed for an increased duration of activity — it's an absolute requirement that you perform your anaerobic cross training with a level of effort that is as high as possible.

In determining whether or not your effort is anaerobic, the time that you take to complete the activity is more critical than the distance that you travel. As an example, suppose two individuals with different levels of fitness each ran 440 yards as fast as possible. The person with the higher fitness level may have run the distance in one minute while the person with the lower fitness level may have needed two minutes. So, the distance run by the two

Left: Many sports and activities are composed of brief, powerful movements that rely heavily upon your anaerobic abilities. (Photo by Larry French)

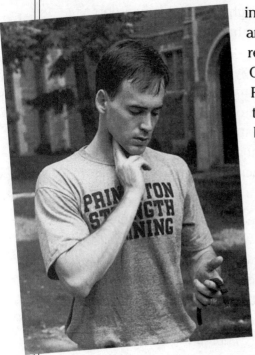

individuals is the same but the different amounts of time taken to perform the activity resulted in the use of different energy sources: One minute of all-out effort involves the ATP-PC System and Anaerobic Glycolysis while two minutes of all-out effort utilizes Anaerobic Glycolysis and the Aerobic System.

Nevertheless, it's often more practical to consider distances when performing anaerobic cross training. If a 3-minute threshold is used as the maximum anaerobic time-limit, you can easily determine a range of distances for your anaerobic cross training. For example, in three minutes most people in reasonably good condition can run about one-half mile. On the other end of the energy continuum, your ATP-PC System can be effectively targeted by all-out efforts that last a handful of seconds or less per repetition — which correlates to running distances of up to about 50 yards. (You can determine a precise range of distances for your anaerobic efforts during running, swimming, rowing and other cross-training activities based upon these time frames and your personal level of fitness.)

Because of its intense nature, most people should only perform anaerobic cross training once or twice a week. Elite or highly competitive athletes may opt for greater frequency. In this case, the number of anaerobic workouts is dependent upon the duration of your efforts. Long- and middle-duration anaerobic efforts of 1.5 - 3.0 minutes (e.g., running between about 440 - 880 yards) can be done 2 - 3 days per week; short-duration anaerobic efforts of less than 90 seconds (e.g., running about 440 yards or less) can be performed 3 - 4 workouts per week. If you reach a point where you are no longer making improvements, then you're probably performing too many anaerobic workouts.

MEANINGFUL ANAEROBIC EXERCISE

After a period of time, you'll likely notice that the same anaerobic cross-training workout — which was originally challenging — can be done with

Above: You can customize the duration of your rest interval by using your heart rate to determine when you're physiologically ready to begin your next work interval. (Photo by Matt Brzycki)

less effort. Therefore, it's critical that you make your anaerobic cross-training activities progressively more difficult in order for you to produce further improvements in your anaerobic fitness.

To ensure that you derive continual anaerobic improvements, you can progressively overload your anaerobic systems by (1) covering the same distances at a faster pace (i.e., in a shorter amount of time); (2) decreasing the length of your recovery intervals; or (3) gradually increasing the distances and decreasing the length of your recovery intervals. For instance, suppose as part of your workout you swam a series of four 100-yard sprints in an average time of 1:30 and took an average recovery time of 3:00 between your efforts. In a future anaerobic workout, you should try to either swim the four 100s in an average time of less than 1:30, take an average recovery time of less than 3:00 between the four 100s or swim the 100s in an average time of a little less than 1:30 and take an average recovery time of slightly less than 3:00 between your efforts. Either way, you caused your anaerobic systems to work harder than they were accustomed to working.

Because of this, it's important for you to keep accurate records of your anaerobic cross-training performances. Maintaining records of your key program components allows you to monitor your progress thereby making your workouts more productive and more meaningful. During anaerobic cross training, the primary program components to keep track of include your training distances, the time of your efforts, the recovery time taken between your efforts and the frequency of your training.

METHODS OF ANAEROBIC CROSS TRAINING

Several different techniques can be used to develop your anaerobic pathways. Remember that the time and intensity (i.e., your exercising heart rate) parameters must be satisfied in order for your activity to be considered anaerobic. For instance, pedaling against a heavy resistance using an all-out effort or swimming laps as fast as possible is necessary to develop your anaerobic pathways.

For the sake of simplicity, most of the ensuing discussions of anaerobic cross training use running as the example. However, all of the methods used in running can be applied to virtually any cross-training activity as well as any type of equipment. For example, if your goal is to run six 440-yard sprints in 90 seconds per sprint, you could simply cycle, row or do another activity with an all-out effort for 90 seconds a total of six times. Incidentally, this also applies to aerobic cross training. If your goal is to run three miles in 24 minutes, you could cycle, row or do another activity for 24 minutes within your heart-rate training zone. Remember, any method that is used to target your anaerobic systems can also be used to challenge your Aerobic System.

If you are an athlete preparing for a specific event — such as rowing or cycling — the best activities to do are the ones you're going to perform in competition. If you want to become a better rower, you must primarily row; if you want to become a better cyclist, you must primarily cycle. Therefore, the best method of anaerobic cross training for sports or activities that involve running — like soccer or basketball — is running. You can — and should — use other cross-training activities to minimize the stress of running but you must run during the majority of your workouts in order to run effectively. An athlete might be in excellent condition to perform a non-weightbearing activity like rowing or cycling but not to do a weightbearing activity like running. (Cross-training options are detailed in Chapter 10.)

If you're a competitive athlete, your workouts should approximate the specific nature of your sport or activity. Anaerobic cross training should be sport-specific — the actual times and distances of your efforts should be based upon the requirements of your sport or activity. For example, if your sport or activity involves a series of intense efforts that are 30 yards or less, then these specific distances should receive the most emphasis during your anaerobic cross training. However, your efforts should also consist of times and distances that are beyond those normally encountered in competition.

Lastly, remember that your Aerobic System provides underlying support for your anaerobic efforts. Therefore, you should develop a strong aerobic foundation before attempting anaerobic cross training.

Interval Training

Structured interval training has been around since the 1930s and has been especially popular among runners and swimmers. However, the principles of interval training can be applied to virtually any cross-training activity.

Essentially, interval training is a series of repeated segments or "intervals" of intense activity (e.g., sprinting) alternated with recovery periods of complete rest or reduced activity. An example of this technique is running a given distance at an intended pace, recovering and then repeating the run-rest program until your workout is completed.

Interval training allows you to reach and sustain a high level of intensity repeatedly for a cumulative time that is greater than what you could achieve during continuous exercise at the same intensity. The reason for this is because the rest intervals allow your anaerobic energy system(s) to partially recover thereby permitting you to make a physiological comeback between your work intervals. Dividing your workout into short, intense efforts with intervals of rest interspersed between consecutive efforts allows you to perform a greater volume of work at the same intensity. So, with an appropriate amount of recovery between your anaerobic efforts, you can run a series of six 440-yard sprints at a pace that might otherwise completely exhaust you after two or three consecutive 440s without a recovery period.

An interval program consists of seven different components which you can manipulate to effectively overload your anaerobic energy systems. All seven of these elements are dependent upon your level of fitness — someone who has a low level of fitness won't be able to perform as much volume as someone who has a high level of fitness. These seven variables are:

1. The number of repetitions.

One variable to consider during interval training is the number of anaerobic efforts — or repetitions — you perform. For instance, you might do eight repetitions of a specified distance during your workout.

2. The training distance.

A second variable during interval training is the distance or the length of the high-intensity work effort — such as running or swimming 200 yards in a specified time. An interval training workout usually begins with long-distance anaerobic efforts and tapers down to shorter efforts.

If you're an athlete interested in improving your anaerobic fitness to better prepare yourself for competition, the length of your work intervals should approximate the requirements of your sport or activity.

3. The work interval.

The intended time of your anaerobic effort is known as the work interval. For instance, your goal might be to row a specified distance in 30 seconds.

4. The rest interval.

The time allotted for recovery between your anaerobic efforts (i.e., the work intervals) is known as the rest (or recovery) interval. It's important for you to receive a sufficient amount of recovery between your anaerobic efforts. This allows your depleted anaerobic energy system(s) sufficient time to recover so that you can make another all-out effort. As an example, the period between your anaerobic work might provide 90 seconds of recovery.

Work/Time (sec)	Distance (yds)	Work: Rest Ratio
0-30	0-220	1:4 to 1:3
30-90	220-440	1:3 to 1:2
90-180	440-880	1:2 to 1:1

Note: The time ranges apply to both the highly and poorly conditioned; the running distances are for those in reasonably good condition.

Table 5.1: Summary of Times, Running Distances and Work: Rest Ratios

The duration of your rest interval is related to the time that it takes you to complete your anaerobic work. You can customize the duration of your rest interval by using your heart rate to determine when you're physiologically ready to begin your next work interval. For example, you might begin your next work interval when your heart rate drops to a predetermined level such as 60 percent of your age-predicted maximum heart rate. An appropriate decrease in heart rate depends upon several factors including the length of the work interval and your level of fitness.

 Your rest interval can consist of either complete inactivity or involve low-intensity activities such as slow walking or easy jogging. Generally, the more intense the work interval, the less intense the rest interval. (Complete inactivity allows your ATP-PC System the opportunity to recover. Performing mild work during the recovery interval inhibits or partially blocks complete restoration of your ATP-PC System. This places greater demands upon your other anaerobic energy system: Anaerobic Glycolysis.)

Incidentally, most sports and activities have built-in recovery intervals because of their intermittent nature. Though these inherent respites are unofficial, unscientific and unpredictable, they produce a fairly successful replenishment of your all-important ATP stores.

5. The work:rest ratio.

The rest interval is usually expressed in relation to the work interval. This is known as the "work:rest ratio" and is most often designated as 1:1, 1:2, 1:3 or 1:4. These ratios state that you should rest either one, two, three or four times the duration that it took you to perform anaerobically. As a general rule, the shorter the duration of your effort — and the higher the intensity — the greater the work:rest ratio. Because of the high level of intensity, any anaerobic effort that you complete in less than 30 seconds requires at least a 1:3 work:rest ratio. As an example, an all-out effort that takes you 20 seconds to perform should be followed by a rest interval of 60 seconds or slightly longer. Anaerobic work done in 30 - 90 seconds needs between a 1:3 and 1:2 work:rest ratio. Finally, performing anaerobically for 90 - 180 seconds requires between a 1:2 and 1:1 work:rest ratio. A summary of times, running distances for those in reasonably good condition and their accompanying work:rest ratios is shown in Table 5.1.

6. The workout distance.

The sum of all the distances performed in your interval workout is the workout distance. With long- and middle-duration anaerobic efforts lasting between 1.5 - 3.0 minutes, the total distance of your workout should not exceed about 2.0 - 2.5 miles (or 3,520 - 4,400 yards) of running; when using anaerobic efforts of less than 90 seconds, the total distance of your workout should not exceed about 1.5 - 2.0 miles (or 2,640 - 3,520 yards) of running. (As a rule of thumb, swimming distances equate to roughly 20 percent of running distances.)

7. The frequency of interval workouts.

A final variable to consider is the frequency of your interval training. Except for elite athletes, interval training should not be performed more than once or twice a week because of the high level of intensity that is required.

An individual interval workout can be written in shorthand. In the language of interval training, a workout written as "8 x 110 yds (0:16/0:48)" indicates that you are to perform eight 110-yard work intervals and that each effort should be done in 16 seconds with a rest interval of 48 seconds between each of the eight repetitions. (Note that the work:rest ratio is 1:3 because each effort is less than 30 seconds in duration.)

Table 5.2 is a detailed example of a nine-week interval program for running that has an anaerobic emphasis. It should be noted again that interval training designed for running can be easily adapted to virtually any type of activity such as swimming, cycling and stair climbing.

Fartlek Training

Fartlek training is thought to be the predecessor of interval training. Originally developed by the Swedes, fartlek training was introduced to the United States in the 1940s. The Swedes are famous in physical education circles for developing systems of training that were basic in structure and used the outdoors as much as possible. As such, fartlek training is usually performed outside over natural but varied terrain that ranges from flat surfaces to steady inclines. For this reason, fartlek training was probably a precursor of

Week	Sprint Reps	Distance (yds)	Work: Rest Ratio	Work Time	Rest Time	Workout Distance	Workouts per Week
1	4	880	1:1	2:35	2:35	3520	1
2	3	880	1:1	2:30	2:30	3520	1
	2	440	1:2	1:15	2:30		
3	2	880	1:1	2:30	2:30	3520	1
	4	440	1:2	1:15	2:30		
4	1	880	1:1	2:25	2:25	3520	1
	6	440	1:2	1:15	2:30		
5	4	440	1:2	1:10	2:20	2640	2
	4	220	1:3	0:35	1:45		
6	3	440	1:2	1:05	2:10	2640	2
	4	220	1:3	0:34	1:42		
	4	110	1:3	0:17	0:51		
7	2	440	1:2	1:05	2:10	2640	2
	6	220	1:3	0:34	1:42		
	4	110	1:3	0:16	0:48		
8	1	440	1:2	1:05	2:10	2640	2
	6	220	1:3	0:33	1:39		
	8	110	1:3	0:16	0:48		
9	1	440	1:2	1:05	2:10	2640	2
	4	220	1:3	0:33	1:39		
	8	110	1:3	0:15	0:45		
	8	55	1:4	0:07	0:28		

Table 5.2: Sample Nine-Week Interval Program for Running

the hill training that is frequently used by modern runners. Fartlek training can also be done indoors using a wide variety of equipment.

Sometimes referred to as "speed play," fartlek training is quite similar to interval training. In structure, fartlek training is less formal and less exact than interval training. Nonetheless, fartlek training achieves anaerobic improvements by using different combinations of effort levels such as walking, jogging and running. The work and rest intervals are left entirely up to the individual — you can change your pace and recover at your own discretion. So, there is definitely an emphasis on "playing" with speed. A sample fartlek workout for running that emphasizes your anaerobic systems might look as follows:

1. jog 440 yards

2. walk 220 yards

3. alternate sprinting 220 yards and walking 220 yards for ten minutes

4. walk 440 yards

5. alternate sprinting 100 yards uphill and walking 100 yards downhill for six minutes

6. walk 440 yards

7. alternate sprinting 50 yards and walking 50 yards for three minutes

Acceleration Sprinting

An effective technique that is used by competitive runners to increase their running speed is known as acceleration sprinting. However, acceleration sprinting can also be used to increase cycling and swimming speeds. As the name implies, acceleration sprinting is characterized by a gradual increase in your speed until a full, all-out effort is reached. When running, for example, you would begin by jogging, then increase to striding and finally accelerate to sprinting the intended distance or duration. Between intervals of work, your rest interval can consist of either complete inactivity or reduced activity such as walking or easy jogging. Gradually increasing your speed throughout the effort allows you to concentrate on your technique which is important to speed development. Acceleration sprinting also provides a smooth transition towards an all-out sprint, thereby minimizing the potential for a muscle strain or pull. A series of 100-yard acceleration sprints for running might look like this:

1. jog 20 yards, stride 30 yards and sprint 50 yards

2. walk 50 yards and repeat ten times

CONDITIONING vs SKILL IMPROVEMENT

When integrating skill work with your anaerobic cross training, improvement in one area is usually sacrificed for improvement in the other. For instance, sprinting as fast as possible is anaerobic cross training; dribbling a soccer ball is sport-specific skill work. If you combine the two activities — that is, sprinting as fast possible while dribbling a soccer ball — you probably won't obtain maximum improvement in either sprinting or dribbling. If your primary goal is to refine an athletic skill — such as dribbling a soccer ball — you need to address that component separately by performing sport-specific skill drills. Likewise, if your main objective is to enhance your anaerobic abilities, then you must focus on that particular area with all-out efforts of brief duration that are sport-specific. Otherwise, your technique is sacrificed at the expense of your conditioning or your conditioning is compromised in order to perfect your skills.

Obviously, skill work and conditioning are blended together during most athletic contests and these two elements must be as identical and as realis-

Women					
Age	**Low**	**Fair**	**Average**	**Good**	**High**
15-19	<91	92-120	121-151	152-182	183+
20-29	<84	85-111	112-140	141-168	169+
30-39	<64	65-84	85-105	106-125	126+
40-49	<49	50-65	66-82	83-98	99+
50+	<37	38-48	49-61	62-75	76+

Men					
Age	**Low**	**Fair**	**Average**	**Good**	**High**
15-19	<112	113-149	150-187	188-224	225+
20-29	<105	106-139	140-175	176-210	211+
30-39	<84	85-111	112-140	141-168	169+
40-49	<64	65-84	85-105	106-125	126+
50+	<49	50-65	66-82	83-98	99+

Table 5.3: Norms for Margaria-Kalamen Test (From Kalamen 1968; Margaria et al. 1966)

tic to a sport as possible. However, developing the speed to perform particular skills is something different than improving your anaerobic fitness. Indeed, skill training and anaerobic cross training are two different components and, therefore, must be treated separately in order for you to attain maximum benefits in both areas.

MEASURING ANAEROBIC FITNESS

Evaluating anaerobic fitness is rather complicated. The difficulty arises because no single test serves as a reliable indicator of your anaerobic fitness. Your two anaerobic energy sources — the ATP-PC System and Anaerobic Glycolysis — contribute in varying ways to a wide range of efforts that last from less than one second up to about three minutes. To obtain a true picture of your anaerobic fitness, it is necessary to perform several tests across the anaerobic spectrum. Needless to say, measuring an instantaneous effort has plenty of room for error.

There is an inverse relationship between the duration that you can sustain an effort at maximal levels and the power requirements of the effort — the shorter the duration of an all-out effort, the greater the output of power. Therefore, you can estimate your anaerobic fitness by measuring your power output.

In scientific terms, "power" is defined as the amount of work done per unit of time — or work divided by time. In this case, "work" is the application of a force over a distance — or force times distance. For example, if you moved 100 kilograms [kg] a distance of .3 meters [m], you did 30 kilogram-meters [kg-m] of work [100 kg x .3 m = 30 kg-m]. If you performed this effort in .25 seconds [sec], your power output was 120 kg-m/sec [30 kg-m divided by .25 sec equals 120 kg-m/sec].

In a laboratory setting, one of the most popular tests of anaerobic ability is known as the Margaria-Kalinen Power Test. At the start of this test, you are to stand 6 meters in front of a staircase. Initiating movement on your own, you would run up the stairs as fast as possible, stepping on every third step (i.e., taking three steps at a time).

 Your power output during this test can be calculated by multiplying your bodyweight (in kilograms) times the vertical distance between the third and the ninth step (in meters) divided by the time of your effort (to the nearest hundredth of a second). For instance, suppose you weigh 154 pounds and covered a vertical distance of 50 inches in .5 seconds. In this case, your power output would be 177.8 kilogram-meters per second [70 kg times 1.27 m divided by .5 seconds = 177.8 kg-m/sec]. (To convert pounds to kilograms, divide pounds by 2.2; to convert inches to meters, multiply inches by 2.54 and divide by 100.) Table 5.3 lists norms for the Margaria-Kalinen Power Test based upon your age and gender. (Values exceeding 270 kg-/sec have been recorded by professional football players.)

Several field tests have a high correlation with your anaerobic ability of very brief duration. Tests evaluating all-out efforts that last a mere instant include the vertical jump, standing long jump and medicine-ball put. A test of anaerobic ability that is a little farther up the anaerobic time frame is running a 50-yard dash.

Of slightly longer duration is a popular laboratory test known as the Wingate Anaerobic Test — which is basically a 30-second all-out sprint on a stationary cycle. Finally, your overall anaerobic abilities — that is, the effectiveness of your ATP-PC System and Anaerobic Glycolysis — can be inferred from all-out efforts that last 30 - 90 seconds such as running 220 - 440 yards as fast as possible.

The upper end of the anaerobic spectrum is actually about three minutes. However, your Aerobic System begins providing assistance to all-out efforts that are beyond about 90 seconds in duration. Therefore, a valid measurement of your anaerobic abilities should involve efforts of less than 1.5 minutes.

6

Efficient Strength Training

A comprehensive cross-training program should incorporate weight-training activities to improve your muscular fitness. Current societal time constraints encourage most people to seek a program that produces the maximal results in the minimum amount of time. As such, efficiency should be your major consideration in developing your strength-training program.

Science has been unable to determine that one strength-training method is superior to another. Research has only shown that a variety of training methods can be used to increase strength. Increases in strength can also be produced by a variety of equipment. Studies have demonstrated no significant differences in strength improvement between groups using free weights and groups using machines.

Since just about any type of program or equipment can yield favorable results, you must decide what is most practical for you based upon safety and time considerations. You can design an efficient strength-training program with virtually any type of equipment by using the following ten principles:

1. Exercise with an appropriate level of intensity.

In Chapter 3, it was noted that your genetics — that is, your inherited characteristics — are the most important determinant of your response to aerobic and anaerobic cross training. Your genetics are also the most significant factor in determining how you respond to strength training.

Other than your genetics, your intensity is the single most important ingredient that influences your results from strength training. Intensity should not be confused with a percentage of a maximum weight. A simple, non-technical definition of intensity is "your level of effort" or "how hard you work."

Remember, you can control your level of intensity when you exercise: Your efforts can be as easy or as difficult as you want. However, the harder you exercise, the better your response. In the weight room, a high level of intensity is characterized by performing each exercise to the point of concentric muscular fatigue or muscular "failure": when you've exhausted your muscles to the extent that you literally cannot raise the weight for any additional repetitions. (Concentric and eccentric muscle contractions are detailed in Chapter 2.)

Failure to reach a desirable level of intensity — or muscular fatigue — will result in submaximal gains in muscular strength. Evidence for this "threshold" is suggested in the scientific literature by the Overload Principle. This principle states that in order for you to increase your muscular strength, your muscles must be stressed — or "overloaded" — with a workload that is beyond their present capacity. Your level of effort must be great enough to exceed this threshold so that a sufficient amount of muscular fatigue is produced to trigger a long-term adaptation: muscular growth. Given proper nourishment and an adequate amount of recovery between workouts, your muscles adapt to those demands by increasing in size and strength. The degree to which this "compensatory adaptation" occurs then becomes a function of your genetics.

So, exercise that doesn't produce enough stress (i.e., muscle fatigue) won't stimulate muscular adaptation. Indeed, a large amount of low-intensity exercise doesn't necessarily create an overload. Exercise that produces too much stress won't permit muscular adaptation either — and may even produce a loss in size and strength. For instance, if you used a hammer on a regular basis for short periods of time you'd form calluses on your palm. Basically, the calluses are a protective adaptation to frictional heat. However, if you hammered for a long enough period of time you'd develop blisters instead. In this case, the excessive demands have surpassed the adaptive ability of your tissue because the stress was too much and too frequent.

It's also important to understand that an inverse relationship exists between time and intensity: As the time or the length of an activity increases, the level of intensity decreases. Stated otherwise, you cannot possibly exercise with an appropriate level of intensity for a long period of time. Here's an analogy: Suppose you were to sprint 440 yards as fast as possible. Depending upon your level of conditioning, your time would probably be in the neighborhood of 60 - 90 seconds. In this instance, your level of intensity was extremely high but the duration of your effort was relatively low. On the other hand, imagine you were to run that same 440-yard distance in two or three minutes. Relative to the first scenario, the duration of your effort was greater but your intensity was lower. As the time of your activity goes up, your level of intensity must go down.

The fact is that you can exercise for a short period of time with a high level of intensity or a long period of time with a low level of intensity. However, you cannot possibly exercise with a high level of intensity for a long period of time. In order to exercise with a fairly high level of intensity, you must train for a relatively brief period of time. If you lengthen the duration of your workout — by increasing either the number of sets or exercises that you normally perform — you must reduce your level of intensity. And, of course, a lower level of intensity is undesirable.

The main reason why most people fail to realize their strength and muscular potential is simply because they don't exercise with an appropriate level of intensity. Clearly, a high level of intensity is an absolute requirement for achieving optimal gains in muscular fitness. Nevertheless, you must also use your judgment in deciding what intensity is suitable for you. Intensity is a relative term that depends upon the current level of fitness and the perception of each individual. Exercise viewed as low-intensity by an active person could be perceived as being high-intensity by a sedentary individual. Therefore, if you haven't been working out on a regular basis or aren't in the best of shape then you should adjust your level of effort accordingly.

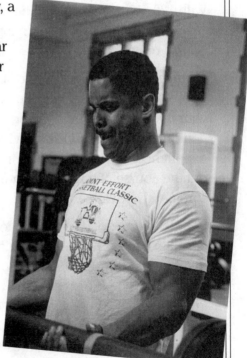

In addition, some people may not be comfortable exercising to the point of muscular exhaustion. If you feel uneasy

Right: A high level of intensity is an absolute requirement for achieving optimal gains in muscular fitness. (Photo by Matt Brzycki)

exercising with a high level of intensity, you can terminate the movements a few repetitions short of complete muscle fatigue. In short, exercise should only be as intense as you feel comfortable.

Simply, a submaximal effort yields submaximal results. The fact that your results from strength training are directly related to your level of effort shouldn't come as much of a surprise. It's like anything else in life: How hard you work at your other cross-training activities, your job and even your relationships largely determines your success at those endeavors.

2. Attempt to increase the resistance used or the repetitions performed every workout.

Unfortunately, little of what is done in most weight rooms can be character-ized as being progressive. It's not uncommon to hear of someone who performs the same number of repetitions with the same amount of weight over and over again, workout after workout. Suppose that today you did a set of leg curls for 10 repetitions with 100 pounds and a month later you're still doing 10 repetitions with 100 pounds. Did you increase your strength? Probably not. On the other hand, what if you were able to do 11 repetitions with 120 pounds a month later? In this case, you performed 10-percent more repetitions with 20-percent more weight — excellent progress over the course of one month.

Changes in the functional and structural abilities of your muscles depend upon the continued application of the Overload Principle. This means that your muscles must be stressed with progressively harder work if they are to continually increase in size and strength. For this reason, your muscles must experience a workload that is increased steadily and systematically through-out the course of your strength-training program. This is often referred to as "progressive overload."

In order to overload your muscles, every time you work out you must at-tempt to increase either the weight you use or the repetitions you perform in relation to your previous workout. This can be viewed as a "double progres-sive" technique (i.e., resistance and repetitions). Stated otherwise, you must impose demands upon your muscles that they haven't previously experi-enced. Exposing your muscles to progressively greater demands stimulates compensatory adaptation in response to the unaccustomed workload.

In brief: If you reach concentric muscle fatigue within your prescribed repetition range — say you did 18 repetitions and your range is 15 - 20 — you should repeat the weight for your next workout and try to improve upon the number of repetitions you did. If you attain or surpass the maximum number of prescribed repetitions in an exercise — say you did 16 repetitions and your range is 10 - 15 — you should increase the resistance for your next workout.

Your progressions in resistance need not be in Herculean leaps and bounds . . . but the weight you use must always be demanding. You should increase the resistance in an amount with which you are comfortable. Your muscles respond better if the progressions in resistance are five-percent or less — depending upon the degree to which the exercise was challenging. For example, suppose that an exercise has a repetition range of 15 - 20. If you barely managed to do 20 repetitions, then you should make a slightly smaller progression in resistance than if you reached muscular exhaustion at 21 or 22 repetitions.

When you make smaller progressions, your muscles hardly notice the slightly heavier weight and your repetitions won't decline much if at all. In other words, it's much easier for your muscles to adapt to subtle increases in resistance than larger ones. As an example, imagine that an exercise has a repetition range of 15 - 20 and you did 200/20 (200 pounds/20 repetitions). If you make a 10-percent increase in resistance the next time you do that exercise (i.e., to 220 pounds), you'll probably notice the heavier weight and it could result in a performance of 220/16. In this scenario, before you can make your next progression in resistance you must improve the number of repetitions you did by 25-percent (from 16 to 20) — which may prove to be a very difficult task. Conversely, if you originally increased the weight by only 2.5 pounds (i.e., to 202.5 pounds), it isn't likely you'll detect the slightly heavier weight and you'd probably get 202.5/20. Another 2.5-pound increase the next time you do that exercise may result in 205/20. Eventually, you might progress to the point where you're doing 220/19. Compared to the previous example, it took you a few more weeks to reach 220 pounds but you allowed your body to adapt gradually. And now, you only need to increase your repetitions by one — from 19 to 20 — to make your next progression in weight.

To make slight progressions in resistance, you can use smaller "Olympic" plates on free-weight movements and plate-loaded machines. Smaller plates are made that weigh as little as 1.25 and 2.5 pounds. If lighter plates aren't available, you can simply hang something from the bar (or movement

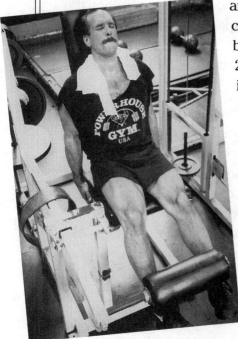

arm) like a small ankle weight. Ankle weights can also be used to make progressions in dumbbell exercises. Making a progression from 20- to 25-pound dumbbells represents a 25-percent increase in resistance. Instead of making such a large percentage increase, you can use the 20-pound dumbbells and put 1.25-pound ankle weights around your wrists. In effect, you'd be using 21.25 pounds — a more reasonable progression in weight of 6.25-percent.

Most selectorized machines have self-contained weight stacks with plates that usually weigh 10, 12.5, 15, 20 or 25 pounds. When using selectorized machines, you can make smaller progressions by using saddle plates — or "add-on" weights — which can be 1.25 or 2.5 pounds. (MedX selectorized machines have a unique compound weight stack that enables the user to make progressions in 2-pound increments without having to use or search for saddle plates.) If saddle plates aren't available, you can take an Olympic plate and secure it to the weight stack by first inserting a selector pin through the hole in the Olympic plate and then into one of the selectorized plates. This is often referred to as "pinning" an Olympic plate to the weight stack. You can also place any object that weighs about 1 or 2 pounds on top of a weight stack — as long as it won't fall off while you're using the equipment.

Again, the resistance you use must always be challenging. If you're just beginning a strength-training program or you change the exercises in your routine, it may take you several workouts before you find a challenging weight. That's okay — simply continue to make progressions in the resistance as needed.

Progressive overload has always been and will always be of utmost importance in achieving physical potential. The bottom line is you must place a demand on your muscles that is beyond what they're accustomed. If you did

Above: The most efficient program is one that produces the maximum possible results in the least amount of time. (Photo by Matt Brzycki)

Right: After raising the weight, you should pause briefly in the position of full muscle contraction of the "mid-range" position. (Photo by Matt Brzycki)

200 pounds today for 12 repetitions, then your next workout you either must attempt to do more repetitions or increase the weight.

3. Perform one set of each exercise to the point of muscular exhaustion.

If performed properly, traditional multiple-set routines (i.e., more than one set) can be effective in overloading your muscles. Multiple-set programs have been used successfully by competitive weightlifters and bodybuilders for decades. And, since many strength and fitness professionals have competed in weightlifting meets and bodybuilding competitions, it's no surprise that traditional multiple-set routines are often prescribed for most people.

In seeking the most efficient strength-training method, a necessary question you must ask is: Can performing one set of each exercise with a high level of intensity give me the same results as performing two or three sets? The answer is a resounding yes. Recall that in order for your muscles to increase in size and strength, they must experience a certain level of fatigue or exhaustion. It's that simple. It really doesn't matter whether your muscles are fatigued in one set or several sets — as long as a sufficient level of fatigue is produced. When performing multiple sets — assuming the weights used are challenging — the cumulative effect of each successive set makes deeper inroads into your muscles thereby creating muscular fatigue; when performing a single-set-to-exhaustion, the cumulative effect of each successive repetition makes deeper inroads into your muscles thereby creating muscular fatigue.

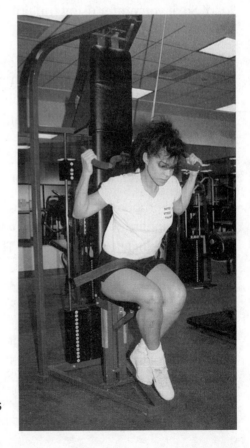

An overwhelming amount of research has shown that one set of an exercise can produce significant strength improvements. Other studies have demonstrated that there are no significant differences between either one, two or three sets of an exercise. Clearly, performing one set to the point of fatigue is a popular and very effective method of strength training that has been advocated by numerous strength and fitness authorities since the early 1970s. Of course, if a single set of an exercise is to be productive, the set must be done with an appropriate level of intensity (i.e., to the point of concentric muscular fatigue). Your muscles must be completely fatigued at the end of each exercise.

If doing one set of an exercise produces the same results as two or three sets, then a one-set protocol represents a more efficient means of strength training. After all, why perform several sets when similar results can be obtained from one set in a fraction of the time?

This is not to say that traditional multiple-set programs are unproductive — but there are several potential problems with such programs. First of all, many people don't do multiple sets properly. Simply doing multiple sets does not guarantee that you've created enough muscle fatigue. If the weights you use aren't demanding enough then you won't create sufficient muscle fatigue and your workout won't be maximally effective. Remember, a large amount of low-intensity work doesn't necessarily produce an overload. So, if you prefer using multiple sets, at least make sure you're challenging your muscles.

 Performing too many sets can also create a situation in which your muscles are broken down in such an extreme manner that your body is unable to regenerate muscle tissue (essentially the resynthesis of myofibrillar proteins). More importantly, doing multiple sets can significantly increase your risk of incurring an overuse injury — such as tendinitis and bursitis — due to repetitive muscular trauma. Finally, multiple sets are extremely inefficient in terms of time and, therefore, are undesirable for time-conscious individuals.

You should emphasize the quality of work done in the weight room rather than the quantity of work. Don't do meaningless sets in the weight room — make every single exercise count. The most efficient program is one that produces the maximum possible results in the least amount of time.

4. Reach concentric muscular exhaustion within a prescribed number of repetitions or amount of time.

Your muscles must be exercised for a certain amount of time with an appropriate level of intensity in order for them to increase in size and strength. Optimal time frames are about 90 - 120 seconds for your hips/buttocks, 60 - 90 seconds for your legs and 40 - 70 seconds for your upper torso. The muscles of your lower body should be exercised for a slightly longer duration because of their greater size and work capacity. (Because it is usually characterized by such short-term, high-intensity efforts, strength training is considered to be an anaerobic endeavor.)

It's usually not practical for you to perform a set for a precise amount of time. However, you can use these optimal time frames to formulate repetition ranges. For instance, if you raise a weight in about 2 seconds and lower it in about 4 seconds, each repetition would be approximately 6 seconds long. Dividing 6 seconds into the time frames that were previously noted yields the following repetition ranges: 15 - 20 for your hips/buttocks, 10 - 15 for your legs and about 8 - 12 for your upper body. Remember, these repetition ranges are based upon a 6-second repetition. The so-called Super Slow Protocol recommends that you raise a weight in 10 seconds and lower it in about 5 seconds (provided that the exercise does not have a significant amount of mechanical friction.) As such, a "Super Slow" repetition is about 15 seconds long. Dividing 15 seconds into the time frames that were mentioned earlier results in the following repetition ranges: 6 - 8 for your hips/ buttocks, 4 - 6 for your legs and about 3 - 5 for your upper torso.

It should be noted that attempting a one-repetition maximum or performing low-repetition movements that are considerably less than those dictated by the optimal time frames increases your risk of injury. Likewise, as an exercise exceeds the recommended time frames, it becomes a greater test of your aerobic endurance rather than your muscular strength.

The repetition ranges that are based upon a 6-second repetition work well for most of the population. However, slightly higher repetition ranges are suggested for the following populations: pregnant females, younger teenagers, older adults, hypertensive individuals and those with orthopedic problems. Slightly higher repetition ranges might be 20 - 25 for exercises involving the hips/buttocks, 15 - 20 for the legs and 10 - 15 for the upper torso. These higher repetition ranges necessitate using somewhat lighter weights which reduces the orthopedic stress placed upon the bones, joints and connective tissue.

Other people — because of their genetic make-up — may also require a slightly higher repetition range. For example, some individuals inherit a higher percentage of slow twitch (ST) muscle fibers than the average person. These individuals would probably benefit more from strength training by performing slightly higher repetitions — like those suggested in the previous paragraph — because their high percentage of ST fibers are more suited for endurance. Conversely, some people inherit a high percentage of fast twitch (FT) fibers which limit their endurance. Slightly lower repetition ranges of perhaps 10 - 15 for the hips/buttocks, 9 - 12 for the legs and 6 - 10 for the upper body would probably produce a better response for someone with a predominance of FT fibers in those body parts.

The only way to positively determine your fiber-type distribution is by removing a small section of your muscle by way of a biopsy and analyzing the tissue sample under a microscope. Most people are understandably reluctant to part with samples of their muscle tissue. However, you can make a logical guesstimate of your fiber-type make-up based upon performance variables. If you're successful at sports or activities that require muscular endurance, you've probably inherited a high percentage of ST muscle fibers and should use slightly higher repetitions. Similarly, if you're proficient at sports or activities requiring strength, speed and/or power, you've likely inherited a high percentage of FT muscle fibers and should perform slightly lower repetitions.

One final point about FT and ST fibers: The use of lower repetitions isn't recommended to convert ST fibers to FT fibers. Likewise, the use of higher repetitions isn't suggested to convert FT fibers to ST fibers. Conversion of fibers appears to be impossible in humans. Performing different repetition ranges is done to maximize your response based upon your already-established predominant muscle fiber type.

5. Perform each repetition with proper technique.

A quality program begins with a quality repetition. Indeed, the most basic and integral aspect of your strength-training program is a repetition. A repetition consists of raising the weight to the mid-range position, pausing briefly and then returning the weight to the starting/stretched position. A repetition is also performed over the greatest possible range of motion (ROM) that is orthopedically safe.

Most people have no understanding or pay little attention to how they perform their repetitions. Remember, unproductive repetitions lead to unproductive sets. Unproductive sets lead to unproductive workouts. And unproductive workouts basically mean that you won't achieve your physical potential.

So, it all comes down to how you do each repetition. A quality repetition starts with the raising of the weight. You should raise the resistance in a deliberate, controlled manner without any jerking movements. Raising a weight in a rapid, explosive fashion is ill-advised for two reasons. First of all, raising a weight with a rapid speed of movement introduces momentum into the movement which makes the exercise less productive and less efficient. After the initial explosive movement, little or no resistance is encountered by your muscles throughout the remaining ROM. In simple terms, the weight is practically moving under its own power. Secondly, raising a weight with a rapid speed of movement exposes your muscles, bones and connective tissue to potentially dangerous forces which magnify the likelihood that you will incur an injury while strength training. Common sense suggests that the faster you lift a weight the more dangerous it becomes. Raising the weight in about 1 - 2 seconds guarantees that you are exercising in a safe, efficient manner.

After raising the weight, you should pause briefly in the position of full muscle contraction or the "mid-range" position. Most people are very weak in the mid-range of exercises because they rarely, if ever, emphasize that position. Pausing momentarily in this position allows you to focus attention on your muscles when they are fully contracted. Further, a brief pause in the mid-range position permits a smooth transition between the raising and the lowering of the weight and helps eliminate the effects of momentum. If you can't pause briefly in the mid-range position, then you probably threw the weight into position by raising it too quickly.

Your eccentric strength is always greater than your concentric strength. Stated otherwise, you can always lower more weight eccentrically than you can raise concentrically. Therefore, it stands to reason that the eccentric portion of the repetition should be emphasized longer than the concentric portion. You should lower the weight back to the starting/stretched position in about 3 - 4 seconds. The lowering of the weight should also be emphasized because it makes the exercise more efficient: The same muscles that you use to raise the weight concentrically are also used to lower it eccentrically — at least with conventional equipment. The only difference is that when you raise a weight, your muscles are shortening against the load and when you lower a weight, your muscles are lengthening against the load. When doing a bicep curl with a barbell, for example, your biceps are used when the weight is raised and your biceps are also used when the weight is lowered. So, lowering the weight represents one half of the entire repetition. If you don't accentuate the eccentric part of the repetition, you'll reduce the efficiency of the exercise by at least 50-percent. By emphasizing the lowering of a weight, each repetition becomes more efficient and each set becomes more productive. Because a "loaded" muscle lengthens as you lower the weight, accentuating the eccentric portion of the repetition also ensures that the exercised muscle is being stretched properly and safely.

In effect, each repetition would be roughly 4 - 6 seconds in length. Most strength and fitness professionals who are opposed to explosive, ballistic movements in the weight room consider a 4 - 6 second repetition as a general guideline for lifting a weight without momentum. (To a degree, the appropriate speed of movement for a repetition depends upon the ROM of the exercise. Remember, all exercises don't have the same ROM. For instance, the elbow joint normally has a ROM that exceeds 135 degrees during the bicep curl and tricep extension. Conversely, the wrist joint normally has a ROM that is less than 90 degrees during wrist flexion and wrist extension. As such, any exercise with a relatively large ROM should take about 6 seconds per repetition; any exercise with a relatively small ROM might take about 4 or 5 seconds per repetition.)

Finally, a quality repetition is done throughout the greatest possible ROM that is orthopedically acceptable — from a position of full stretch to a position of full muscular contraction and back to a position of full stretch. Exercising throughout a full ROM allows you to maintain (or perhaps increase) your flexibility. Furthermore, it ensures that your entire muscle is being exercised — not just a portion of it — thereby making the movement more efficient. Research has shown that full-range exercise is necessary for a full-range effect.

Remember, how you lift a weight is more important than how much weight you lift. Your strength training will be safer and more efficient by performing each repetition with proper technique.

6. Strength train for no more than one hour per workout.

More may be better when it comes to knowledge and happiness but more isn't necessarily better when it comes to strength training. If you are training with a high level of intensity — and you should — you literally cannot exercise for a long period of time.

It's important to note that carbohydrates are your body's preferred fuel during intense exercise. Carbohydrates circulate in your bloodstream as glucose and are stored in your liver and muscles as glycogen. Most people exhaust their carbohydrate stores after about one hour of intense exercise. For that reason, your strength workouts should be completed in one hour or less. Under normal circumstances, if you are spending much more than one hour in the weight room then you probably aren't exercising with an appropriate level of intensity. This one-hour window of time also dictates the number of sets that you can perform for each exercise.

The exact duration of your workout depends on several factors such as the size of the facility, the amount of available equipment, the preparation for each exercise (i.e., changing plates, moving pins and so on), the number of people in the facility, your transition time between each set, the availability of supervisory personnel and the managerial ability of those personnel. Generally speaking, however, you should be able to complete a productive workout in 60 minutes or less.

The time you take between each exercise or set depends upon your level of fitness. You should begin your next exercise or set as soon as you catch your breath or feel that you can produce a maximal level of effort. As you adjust to the demands of intense exercise and your fitness level improves, you should be able to recover adequately between exercises within 1 - 3 minutes. Doing your strength training with a minimal amount of recovery time between exercises elicits a metabolic conditioning effect that cannot be approached by traditional multiple-set programs. (Metabolic conditioning is detailed in Chapter 7.)

7. Perform no more than about 14 exercises each workout.

For most people, a comprehensive strength-training program can be performed using 14 exercises or less during each workout. The focal point for most of these movements should be your major muscle groups (i.e., your hips/buttocks, legs and upper torso). Include one exercise for your hips/buttocks, hamstrings, quadriceps, calves/dorsi flexors, biceps, triceps, abdominals and lower back. Because your shoulder joint allows movement at many different angles, two movements should be selected for your chest, upper back (your "lats") and shoulders. You should choose any exercises that you prefer in order to train those body parts.

For some individuals, a thorough workout may require slightly more than 14 movements. For instance, if you're involved in a combative sport — such as football, rugby, wrestling, boxing or judo — a comprehensive workout should include an additional 2 - 4 neck exercises to strengthen and protect your cervical area against possible traumatic injury. Additionally, if you participate in a sport or activity that requires grip strength — such as softball, tennis or golf — you should perform one forearm exercise.

Once again, more isn't necessarily better when it comes to strength training. Performing too many movements may produce too much stress, which impedes muscular adaptation. A workout consisting of 20 movements could be metabolically devastating to someone with a low tolerance level for exercise. In addition, the more exercises that you perform, the harder it will be for you to maintain a desirable level of intensity.

Occasionally, you can do an extra movement to emphasize a particular body part. As long as you continue to make improvements in your strength, you aren't performing too many exercises. So, if your workout consists of 20 exercises and you're making progress then you aren't overstressing your system. But if you start to level off or "plateau" in one or more exercises, it's probably due to a catabolic effect from performing too many movements.

8. Whenever possible, exercise your muscles from largest to smallest.

Your strength-training program should begin with exercises that influence your largest muscles and proceed to those that involve your smallest muscles. Exercises for your hips/buttocks should be performed first, followed by your upper legs (hamstrings and quadriceps), lower legs (calves or dorsi flexors), upper torso (chest, upper back and shoulders), arms (biceps, triceps and forearms), abdominals and finally your lower back.

It's important not to fatigue your mid-section early in your workout. Your abdominals stabilize your rib cage and serve as respiratory muscles during intense exercise to facilitate forced expiration. Therefore, early fatigue of your abdominals would detract from your performance in other exercises that involve your larger, more powerful muscles. Your lower back should be the very last muscle that you exercise. Fatiguing your lower back earlier in your workout will also hinder your performance in other movements.

Exercises for your neck musculature may be done at the beginning of your workout or just after your lower-body exercises are completed (i.e., prior to beginning your upper-body movements). This would seem to violate the "largest to smallest" rule. However, at the end of your workout you'll be quite fatigued — physically as well as mentally. Because of this, you'll be less likely to train your all-important neck area with a desirable level of effort or enthusiasm. Exercising your neck earlier in your workout when you're less fatigued elicits a more favorable response.

Your arms should not be exercised before your upper torso. Multiple-joint movements done for your upper body require the use of your arms to assist the movement. Your arms are the "weak link" in the exercise because they

Right: If you're involved in a combative sport, a comprehensive workout should include an additional 2-4 neck exercises to strengthen and protect your cervical area against possible traumatic injury. (Photo by Matt Brzycki)

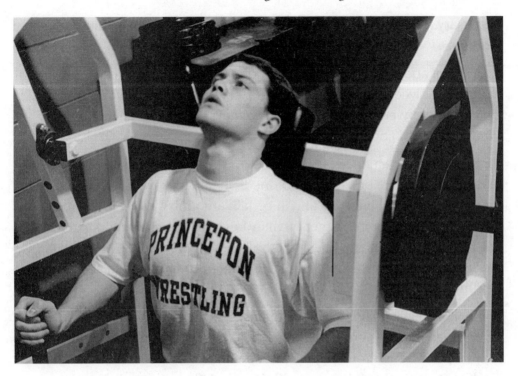

are smaller. So, if you fatigue your arms first, you'll weaken an already weak link, thereby limiting the workload placed on the muscles of your upper torso. Likewise, your legs are the weak link when performing exercises for your hips and buttocks. Consequently, avoid training your legs — especially your quadriceps and hamstrings — before performing an exercise for your hips/buttocks, such as the leg press.

9. Strength train 2 - 3 times per week on non-consecutive days.
Intense strength training places great demands and stress on the muscles. Your muscles must receive an adequate amount of recovery between your strength workouts in order to adapt to those demands.

Adaptation to the stress occurs during the recovery process. Your muscles don't get stronger during your workout — your muscles get stronger while you recover from your workout. When you lift weights, your muscle tissue is broken down and the recovery process allows your muscles time to rebuild themselves. Think of this as allowing a wound to heal. If you had a scab and picked at it every day, you would delay the healing process. However, if you left it alone you would permit the damaged tissue time to heal. There are individual variations in recovery ability — everyone has different levels of tolerance for exercise. However, a period of about 48 - 72 hours is usually necessary for muscle tissue to recover sufficiently from an intense strength workout.

A period of about 48 hours is also required to replenish your depleted carbohydrate (or glycogen) stores. Therefore, it is suggested that you strength train 2 - 3 times per week on non-consecutive days — such as on Monday, Wednesday and Friday.

An appropriate frequency (and volume) of strength training can be likened to doses of medication. In order for medicine to improve a condition, it must be taken at specific intervals and in certain amounts. Taking medicine at a greater frequency or in a larger quantity beyond what is needed can have harmful effects. Similarly, an "overdose" of strength-training — in which workouts are done too often or have too much volume — can also be detrimental.

Some individuals respond well to three weekly workouts; others react more favorably to two sessions per week. (In rare circumstances, an individual may respond better from one workout per week.) In general, you can obtain significant improvements in strength from as little as two weekly workouts. Performing any more than three "doses" of strength training a week can gradually become counterproductive if the demands placed on your muscles have exceeded your recovery ability.

Your muscles begin to progressively lose strength if they aren't exercised within about 96 hours of their previous workout. That's why it's important for an athlete to continue strength training even while in-season or while competing. However, the workouts should be reduced to twice a week due to the increased activity level of practices and competitions. One session should be done as soon as possible following a competition and another no later than 48 hours before the next competition. So, an athlete who competes on Saturdays and Tuesdays should strength train on Sundays and Wednesdays (or Thursdays -- providing that it's not within 48 hours of the next competition). From time to time, an athlete may only be able to strength train once a week because of a particularly heavy schedule such as competing three times in one week or several days in a row.

How do you know if your muscles have had an adequate amount of recovery? You should see a gradual improvement in the amount of weight and/or number of repetitions that you're able to do over the course of several weeks. If not, then you're probably not getting enough recovery between workouts — which could be the result of performing too many sets, too many repetitions or too many exercises.

10. Keep accurate records of your performance.

The importance of accurate record keeping cannot be overemphasized. Records are a log of what you've accomplished during each and every exercise of each and every strength session. In a sense, your workout card is a history of your activities in the weight room.

Many people believe that they don't need a workout card because they can remember their weights and repetitions. In all likelihood, they've probably been doing the same weight and the same repetitions for so long that those numbers have become memorized.

Your workout card can be an extremely valuable tool to monitor your progress and make your workouts more meaningful. Additionally, keeping track of your performance is helpful in identifying exercises in which you've reached a plateau. In the unfortunate event of an injury, you can also gauge the effectiveness of your rehabilitative process if you have a record of your pre-injury strength levels.

A workout card can take an infinite number of appearances and need not be elaborate. However, you should be able to record your bodyweight, the date of each workout, the weight used for each exercise, the number of repetitions performed for each exercise, the order in which the exercises were completed and any necessary seat adjustments.

Your card can list specific exercises and the more common movements (e.g., leg curl, leg extension, bench press) and/or may contain blank spaces so that you can fill in your own menu of exercises. The recommended repetition ranges should also be given for each exercise along with spaces to record any seat adjustments.

7 Metabolic Conditioning

Most people typically perform their strength training separate from their conditioning activities. Yet, many individuals — especially athletes — are required to integrate their muscular strength with their aerobic conditioning.

Metabolic conditioning is essentially a combination of intense strength training (or other anaerobic efforts) and aerobic conditioning. It involves three major biological systems: the musculoskeletal, respiratory and circulatory systems. In order for you to improve your metabolic fitness, these three systems must share the physiological demands.

Unfortunately, conditioning of the metabolic system is rarely emphasized or even addressed. However, a thorough understanding of metabolic conditioning and an application of specific training techniques can enhance your functional fitness.

PROJECT TOTAL CONDITIONING

In the early 1970s, research designated as "Project Total Conditioning" was conducted at the United States Military Academy in New York. The research used members of several athletic teams at the academy as test subjects. Project Total Conditioning actually consisted of a number of different studies. For example, one study examined the effects of a strength-training program on the neck size and strength of rugby players. Another study investigated the effects of two different training protocols on the vertical jumping ability of volleyball players.

However, the main portion of Project Total Conditioning was a 6-week study that examined metabolic conditioning. An experimental group consisted of

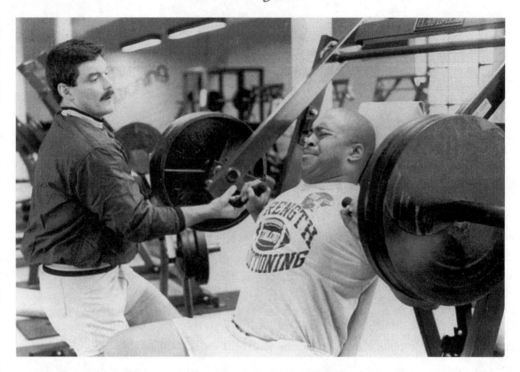

18 varsity football players from the academy (a nineteenth subject was injured during spring football practice). This group performed a strength-training workout three times per week on alternate days with two days rest after the third workout of the week. Each workout consisted of ten exercises and took an average of about 30 minutes to complete. (The subjects also performed six neck exercises twice per week.) Each subject was required to perform as many repetitions as possible using proper technique in every exercise of every workout. One set of each exercise was done to the point of muscular fatigue within a repetition range of 5 - 12. The group took a minimum amount of recovery time between exercises.

In order to minimize the influence of the "learning effect," the experimental group followed the training protocol for two weeks prior to the study. (The "learning effect" refers to the often dramatic increases initially attained by individuals which is attributable to improvement in their neurological functioning not muscular strength.) Prior to the 6-week study, the subjects were pretested in several areas — including body composition, strength, cardiovascular fitness, the 40-yard dash, the vertical jump and flexibility — and were retested following the study.

Above: Your metabolic fitness may be improved by simply performing your strength training with a high level of intensity while taking very little rest between your exercises. (Photo by Rick Phelps)

The study produced very compelling results. After 6 weeks of training, the subjects increased the resistance they used between their first and seventeenth workouts by an average of 58.54%. The minimum improvement in strength was 45.61% while the maximum increase in strength was 69.70%. (Incidentally, the average increase in the resistance that was used between the second and sixteenth workouts was 43.06%.) The subjects also increased the number of repetitions they performed between their first and seventeenth workouts by an average of 6.59%.

Interestingly, the time that the subjects needed to complete their workouts decreased substantially. Comparing the first workout to the seventeenth, the experimental group reduced the average duration of their workouts by 24.09% — from an average of 37.73 minutes to an average of 28.64 minutes. Two individuals almost literally cut their workout times in half — one from 49 to 25 minutes and the other from 43 to 22 minutes — yet increased their strength levels by 68.32% and 65.59%, respectively. A third individual reduced his workout time from 42 to 27 minutes and increased his strength by 66.32%.

Besides the tremendous improvements in muscular strength, the subjects also reduced their average time in the 2-mile run by 88 seconds — from an average of 13:18 to an average of 11:50. This represented an average improvement of 11% — without having performed any running except during the course of spring football practice (which occurred during the first 4 weeks of training). The subjects also had lower resting heart rates following the six weeks of training. In addition, the experimental group had lower exercising heart rates at various workloads on a stationary cycle and they were able to perform more work before reaching heart rates of 170 beats per minute.

At the end of the 6-week study, the experimental group had reduced their average time in the 40-yard dash from 5.1467 seconds to 5.0933 seconds — a 1.04% improvement. Their vertical jump had increased from an average of 22.6 inches to an average of 24.067 inches — an average improvement of 6.49%. Finally, their average improvement in three flexibility measures was 10.92%.

These striking results are even more impressive when you consider that they were accomplished in such a time-efficient manner. In fact, the total amount of actual training time performed by each individual during the 6-week program averaged less than 8.5 hours — which is less than 30 minutes per workout. It should be noted that the test subjects were highly conditioned football players who were already quite strong and fit at the start of the program. Nevertheless, the study demonstrated the effects of short-duration, high-intensity strength training on metabolic conditioning.

TYPES OF METABOLIC WORKOUTS

Your metabolic fitness may be improved by simply performing your strength training with a high level of intensity while taking very little rest between your exercises. Performed in this fashion, the shared demands placed on your major biological systems creates a metabolic conditioning effect that cannot be approached by traditional methods of training. The two most popular types of metabolic workouts are high-intensity training and circuit training.

High-Intensity Training (HIT)

One form of metabolic conditioning that has recently seen a renewed interest is high-intensity training or, simply, HIT. In the early 1970s, Nautilus inventor Arthur Jones popularized the brief, intense strength-training work-outs that would later become known as HIT in the mid-1980s. In recent years, HIT has gradually become increasingly popular among highly competitive male and female athletes in a variety of sports and activities. HIT is currently used by professional athletes in the National Basketball Association (NBA), the National Hockey League (NHL) and Major League Baseball (MLB) as well as nearly one dozen teams in the National Football League (NFL). In addition, HIT is used by thousands of collegiate athletes who participate in virtually every sport imaginable — and the numbers are growing. The United States Women's Basketball Team also used HIT on their way to the 1996 Olympic gold medal.

There are many interpretations and variations of HIT. However, most versions of HIT have several common denominators. As the name implies, HIT is characterized by intense, aggressive efforts — each exercise is typically performed to the point of muscular fatigue or "failure." A minimal number of sets is usually performed — often only one set of each exercise but sometimes as many as three sets. Another characteristic of HIT is the emphasis on progressive overload — whenever possible, an attempt is made to increase either the repetitions that are performed or the resistance that is used from one workout to the next. With safety as a major concern, HIT doesn't include explosive movements or momentum — all repetitions are done with a controlled speed of movement. Additionally, HIT is comprehensive — training all of the major muscle groups is a priority.

In general, HIT also involves very brief workouts with a minimum amount of recovery taken between exercises. The short recovery interval between exercises enables you to maintain a fairly high heart rate for the duration of your workout. Like other forms of metabolic conditioning, the length of the recovery interval taken between exercises depends upon your present level of metabolic fitness. The recovery period isn't structured, timed or predetermined. Initially, however, a recovery time of perhaps three minutes may be necessary between efforts; with improved fitness, your pace should be quickened to the point where you are moving as rapidly as possible between exercises. (These and other HIT concepts are described in greater detail in Chapter 6.)

In short, HIT places an incredible workload upon every major muscle in your body and, at the same time, stresses your circulatory and respiratory pathways. Furthermore, this type of workout can be used to improve your metabolic fitness in a safe and time-efficient manner.

The 3x3 Workout. One of the most strenuous of all HIT workouts is sometimes referred to as a "3x3" (i.e., three by three) and, for this reason, deserves special note. A 3x3 Workout simply means that you do three exercises that are repeated three times. For example, the most popular and demanding version of a 3x3 Workout looks like this: leg press, dip, chin, leg press, dip, chin, leg press, dip and chin. However, this routine is just one of many possible versions of a 3x3 Workout. This form of metabolic conditioning can actually be modified in a countless number of ways. (Detailed information on specific exercises mentioned throughout this chapter can be found in *A Practical Approach to Strength Training* which is published by Masters Press.)

Essentially, a 3x3 Workout consists of a multiple-joint hip movement followed by a multiple-joint chest movement followed by a multiple-joint upper-back movement and repeated two more times with as little rest as possible between exercises. These three types of movements address every major muscle in your body including your hips/buttocks, quadriceps, hamstrings, chest, upper back, shoulders, biceps, triceps and forearms.

The most demanding multiple-joint exercises for your hips/buttocks (along with your quadriceps and hamstrings) are some type of leg press, squat or deadlift (with an Olympic bar, a trap bar or dumbbells). Dips and chins certainly represent the most challenging selections for your chest and upper back, respectively. Those who cannot perform dips and/or chins with their bodyweight can do alternative multiple-joint movements that exercise the same muscles. Any kind of multiple-joint movement that involves a pushing motion — such as the bench press, incline press or push-ups — can be used to influence your chest musculature (as well as your shoulders and triceps). Any type of multiple-joint movement that involves a pulling motion — such as a lat pulldown or seated row — is suitable for targeting the muscles of your upper back (along with your biceps and forearms).

The first time through the three movements, you should reach muscle fatigue at about 20 reps for the hip/buttock exercise, 12 for the chest exercise and 12 for the upper-back exercise. When the sequence is repeated the second time, the repetition goals would be 15 for the hip/buttock exercise, 10 for the chest exercise and 10 for the upper-back exercise. The third time through the movements should have goals of 12 for the hip/buttock exercise, 8 for the chest exercise and 8 for the upper-back exercise. In summary, the repetition goals for these movements should be 20, 15 and 12 for the hip/buttock exercise and 12, 10 and 8 for the chest and upper-back exercises.

A 3x3 Workout is extremely time-efficient — most variations can be performed in about 20 minutes or less. The simplicity of this specific type of HIT workout can be deceptive. Though it may not appear to be demanding, a 3x3 Workout — if done as outlined above — can place a Herculean workload upon your physiological systems that translates into tremendous metabolic stress.

Circuit Training

One of the oldest and most popular forms of metabolic conditioning has been dubbed "circuit training." The birth of circuit training can be traced back to England in the 1950s. With circuit training, the idea is to perform a series of exercises (or activities) in a sequence or "circuit" with a very brief recovery period between each "station." In a sense, therefore, circuit training is a form of interval training. (Chapter 5 discusses interval training as it applies to anaerobic cross training.)

Circuit Weight Training. The merger of circuit training with weight training is known as "circuit weight training" or, simply, CWT. Usually, CWT is performed on a multi-station apparatus — such as a Universal Multi-Gym. There are several advantages in using multi-station equipment for CWT. First of all, the exercises of multi-station equipment are in close proximity to each other which allows you to move quickly around the circuit. Secondly, the selectorized weight stacks of multi-station equipment enable you to make

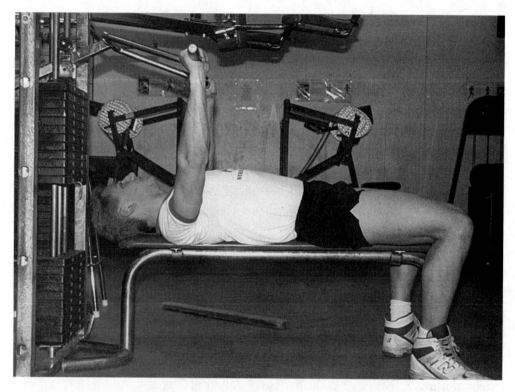

faster and easier adjustments in resistance. Nevertheless, CWT can also be performed with single-station pieces and/or free weights provided that the distance between the equipment isn't too great.

CWT is very versatile — you can manipulate the number of exercises/ stations, the number of repetitions performed and the amount of recovery taken between movements. The number of exercises you do in the circuit and the amount of recovery taken between the exercises is a function of your level of fitness. However, a comprehensive session of CWT involves a series of about 12 - 14 exercises or stations that target each of your major muscle groups. A total-body circuit on a Universal Multi-Gym might be as follows: leg press, leg curl, leg extension, bench press, dip, pull-up, lat pulldown, seated press, shoulder shrug, bicep curl, tricep extension, wrist flexion and sit-up. (Several other productive exercises can be done on most multi-station equipment including the upright row, knee-up and side bend.)

 At each station, you can either perform a given number of repetitions or do as many repetitions as possible during a specified time frame (with a controlled speed of movement). At a pace of 60 seconds per exercise with 30

Above: Circuit weight training is usually performed on a multi-station apparatus — such as a Universal Multi-Gym. (Photo by Matt Brzycki)

seconds of recovery between stations (including the set-up for the next exercise), a circuit of 12 - 14 stations can be completed in as little as 18 - 21 minutes. It should be noted that the resistance you use at each station should permit you to reach muscle fatigue by the end of the allotted exercise time.

To ensure that you obtain continued metabolic improvements from CWT, you can progressively overload your metabolic system by (1) increasing the resistance you use at a given station; (2) increasing the length of the work interval (thereby doing more repetitions); (3) decreasing the length of the recovery interval taken between stations; or (4) any combination of the three previous options.

To summarize CWT: You begin at a particular station and complete one set of an exercise. After this, you move to the next station in the circuit where you set-up for your next exercise and rest for the remainder of your recovery period. This cycle is repeated over and over again until the entire circuit is complete.

Circuit Aerobic Training. In the last few years, there's been a growing interest in circuit aerobic training (CAT) which involves a series of aerobic cross-training activities or stations. The circuit can be designed a number of different ways — you can vary the number of cross-training activities, the duration and intensity of each activity and the amount of recovery taken between stations. Most of these variables are dependent upon your fitness level. Your goal, however, is to perform the equivalent of about 20 - 60 minutes of aerobic activity with an appropriate level of effort. Keep in mind that thirty minutes of exercise can be done as one 30-minute session, two 15-minute sessions, three 10-minute sessions or even six 5-minute sessions. So, you might exercise for 10 minutes on a stationary cycle, 10 minutes on a rower and 10 minutes on a stair-climbing machine for a total of 30 minutes of cross-training activity. Or, you might perform each of those same three activities for 5 minutes but repeat the circuit twice for a total of 30 minutes. Regardless, your level of intensity should be as high as possible during your efforts. (It probably wouldn't be practical — or permissible — for you to monopolize a group of activities for intervals of less than five minutes per station in a commercial facility.)

Other Variations. Yet another version of circuit training is to integrate weight-training exercises with one or more aerobic-training activities. For instance, you might do a strength-training exercise, pedal a stationary cycle for 1 - 3 minutes, do another strength-training exercise, pedal a stationary cycle for another 1 - 3 minutes and so on. Along these lines, a simple but brutal form of metabolic conditioning can be done by alternating dips and chins with running. In other words, you might do a set of dips, run a short distance, do a set of chins, run a short distance and repeat this circuit several times. (If performed indoors, you can run on a motorized treadmill.)

The "Fitness Trail" is a form of circuit training that was originated in several of the Scandinavian countries. This method of circuit training is performed outdoors in a natural environment such as a park. A typical Fitness Trail consists of numerous stations that are positioned several hundred yards apart and arranged along a circuitous route. You would walk, jog or run to a station, stop and perform some type of agility (i.e., hurdles, log walks and vaults), calisthenic (i.e., push-ups, sit-ups, chins, dips) or flexibility exercise and then proceed to the next station.

METABOLIC DYNAMICS

At rest, your body doesn't consume much oxygen and your energy needs are easily satisfied by your Aerobic System. As your metabolic demands increase during exercise, you require more energy immediately. Your Aerobic System cannot transport and deliver oxygen fast enough to address this physiological urgency. Therefore, you must rely upon your anaerobic systems to provide energy until your Aerobic System is able to meet your needs.

For the most part, metabolic conditioning involves all-out efforts that last about 60 - 90 seconds (though the time of activity can approach 120 seconds when performing strength-training exercises for your hips/buttocks). In the early stages of intense exercise, a limited amount of energy can be supplied rapidly by your two anaerobic sources: the ATP-PC System and Anaerobic Glycolysis. During intense efforts, your ATP-PC System exhausts your phosphagen stores in a matter of seconds; as a result of Anaerobic Glycolysis, the glycogen content of your working muscles drops progressively. As additional oxygen becomes available, your Aerobic System is used to a greater degree. After a few minutes, your Aerobic System is able to furnish all the energy needed for mild exercise.

Metabolic conditioning presents an enormous physiological challenge to your musculoskeletal, respiratory and circulatory systems. In response to this metabolic stress, your systems make a number of sudden, temporary adjustments that return to resting levels once you complete your effort. The degree of your metabolic response increases in direct proportion to your intensity and the duration of the activity and is also related to other factors such as your

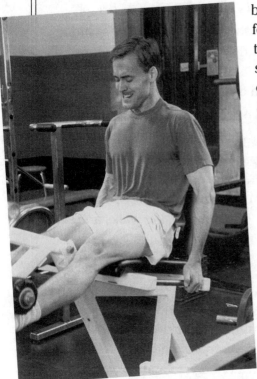

body size, gender and level of fitness. There-fore, detailing your precise biological reaction to general metabolic conditioning is impossible. However, your metabolic adjustments can be estimated with a reasonable degree of accuracy. When going from a resting state to an exercising state, your predicted physiological responses include:

Musculoskeletal Responses

When performing a strength-training exercise, your intensity is lowest during the first repetition. At this point, only a small percentage of your available muscle fibers is recruited (or innervated) by your nervous system — just enough to move the weight. When the muscular intensity is low, your metabolic needs are met by your slow-twitch fiber population. As you do each repetition, your intensity increases progressively and deeper inroads are made into your muscles. Some of your muscle fibers fatigue and are no longer able to keep up with the increasing metabolic demands. Fresh fibers are simultaneously called upon to assist the fatigued fibers in generating ample force. Your fast-twitch fibers are recruited by your nervous system only when your fatigue-resistant slow-twitch fibers have depleted their energy stores and cannot meet the force requirements. This process continues until the last repetition when you reach concentric muscular fatigue and your intensity is at its highest. Now, the collective efforts of your remaining fibers cannot produce enough force to raise the weight. During this final repetition, the cumulative effect of each preceding repetition has fatigued your muscles thereby providing a sufficient — and efficient — stimulus for muscular growth. It should be noted that your first few repetitions are the least productive because your intensity is low. On the other hand, your very last repetition is the most productive because your intensity is very high.

Respiratory Responses

The most obvious respiratory response to intense metabolic activity is an increase in the frequency and depth of your breathing. Indeed, rapid and

Above: During intense exercise, your exercising muscles may receive 85-90 percent of the total blood flow. (Photo by Matt Floyd)

deep breathing is an unmistakable indicator of intense activity. Your labored breathing leads to a heightened sense of respiratory distress, general discomfort and widespread fatigue. Specifically, your number of breaths per minute (breaths/min) may increase from a resting rate of about 10 - 12 breaths/min to about 40 - 50 breaths/min.

Tidal volume refers to the amount of air entering or leaving your lungs during a single breath and is measured in liters per breath (L/breath). During intense activity, your tidal volume may rise to more than six times it's resting level — from about 0.5 L/breath to about 3.0 L/breath or more.

The amount of air you inhale or exhale each minute is known as your pulmonary ventilation. It is measured in liters per minute (L/min) and is calculated by multiplying the frequency of your breathing (in breaths/min) by your tidal volume (in L/breath). Because of the combined increases in your rate and depth of breathing, your pulmonary ventilation may increase from 5 L/min [10 breaths/min x 0.5 L/breath] to more than 150 L/min [50 breaths/min x 3.0 L/breath]. To aid in forced expiration during intense efforts, there is also a greater involvement of your respiratory muscles — that is, your abdominal and internal intercostal muscles (which lie between your ribs). In fact, your respiratory muscles may demand 8 - 10 percent of your oxygen intake during intense exercise.

Circulatory Responses

When you exercise, your heart beats faster to meet the demands of your muscles for more blood and oxygen. Specifically, your heart rate may climb from a resting level of about 60 - 70 beats per minute (bpm) to as much as 80 - 90 percent of your age-predicted maximum or more for brief periods. (Your heart rate actually increases above resting levels prior to your efforts due to the so-called anticipatory response.) The more intense the exercise or activity, the faster your heart beats. The increase in your heart rate is greatest when you perform exercises involving your larger muscle groups — particularly your hips and legs. Monitoring your heart rate during exercise provides a very accurate reflection of the metabolic intensity of the exercise.

Stroke volume refers to the volume of blood pumped by your heart and is measured in liters per beat (L/beat). During intense efforts, your stroke volume may rise from about .08 L/beat to perhaps 0.2 L/beat or more. As a result of the combined increases in your stroke volume and heart rate, your cardiac output may increase from about 5 L/min [e.g., .08 L/beat x 60 bpm] to more than 30 L/min [e.g., 0.2 L/beat x 150 bpm]. Once your stroke volume reaches your physiological limit, further increases in your cardiac output are only possible through increases in your heart rate.

Your cardiac output is distributed to your organs and tissues according to their functions and needs at any given moment. During intense activity, your blood flow is redistributed from areas where it isn't very critical to areas where it is absolutely essential. Specifically, there is a diminished blood flow to your inactive muscles and less active tissues such as your liver, kidneys and digestive organs (i.e., your stomach and intestines). At rest, 15 - 20 percent of your systemic blood flow is to your muscles — the majority of the blood goes to your digestive organs and brain. During intense exercise, your blood flow is redirected to your working muscles. In fact, your exercising muscles may receive 85 - 90 percent of the total blood flow. This means that for a cardiac output of 30 L/min, more than 25 liters of blood can be delivered to your active muscles every minute. Your heart also receives an increased supply of blood during intense efforts — from a resting level of about 0.25 L/min to about 0.75 L/min. (The blood flow to your brain is unchanged.)

Your blood pressure is measured in millimeters of mercury (mmHg). Your systolic blood pressure increases in proportion to your exercise intensity and can rise from a resting level of about 120 mmHg to more than 200 mmHg. During intense activity, the diastolic blood pressure of healthy individuals remains at about 70 mmHg or drops slightly. Maximum blood pressure usually occurs at maximum heart rate.

Your body temperature rises during intense exercise — especially in hot, humid conditions. Your body has a temperature-regulatory mechanism and, like a thermostat, tries to maintain its temperature at a relatively constant value of roughly 98.6 degrees Fahrenheit (or about 37 degrees Celsius). During vigorous activity, your body temperature may exceed 102 degrees Fahrenheit (or about 39 degrees Celsius). As your body temperature rises, there is an increased blood flow from your warmer core to the surface of your skin. This process facilitates heat dissipation and allows heat loss. Unfortunately, this also reduces the amount of blood available to supply your working muscles with oxygen. (Guidelines for exercising in hot, humid environments are given in Chapter 12.)

General Responses

Short-term, high-intensity activity increases the production of carbon dioxide and lactic acid. This, in turn, lowers your pH. Your muscle pH may briefly decrease from a resting value of about 7.0 to as low as 6.4. The lactate spreads from your muscles into the surrounding tissues and eventually spills into your blood. This causes your blood pH to temporarily drop from a resting value of perhaps 7.4 to as low as 6.8. As the lactic acid begins to accumulate, it irritates your nerve endings and causes feelings of muscular pain, discomfort, distress and fatigue. As lactic acid accumulates, it also causes your breathing to become labored.

During intense metabolic conditioning, your oxygen intake may increase from about 3.5 ml/kg/min at rest to about 26.0 ml/kg/min or more. For a 165-pound person, this equates to an increase from a resting level of roughly 0.25 L/min to about 2.0 L/min or more. Compared to pure aerobic cross-training, these oxygen intake values are somewhat low. Such low values are primarily due to the intermittent nature of metabolic conditioning. At any given heart rate, the metabolic demands — in terms of oxygen intake — are lower for strength training compared to aerobic training. Research has shown that the oxygen intake during strength training averages 68% of that seen during aerobic training at the same exercising heart rate. Expressed in different terms: At a given level of oxygen intake, heart rates are higher during strength training compared to aerobic training. For instance, an oxygen intake of 25 ml/kg/min elicits a heart rate of about 180 bpm during strength training compared to a heart rate of about 155 bpm for aerobic training. During strength training, the heart rate is disproportionately elevated relative to oxygen intake.

Your expenditure of calories per minute (cal/min) is also elevated during intense activity. Like most of your other metabolic responses, the rate of your caloric expenditure largely depends upon your intensity and your bodyweight. The rate of caloric expenditure for a 165-pound individual may increase from about 1.3 cal/min to perhaps 10.0 cal/min or more. Finally, it should be noted that your oxygen intake and caloric expenditure is greatest when training the larger muscles in the body such as your hips and legs.

8

Stretching Your Muscles

Flexibility can be defined as the range of motion (ROM) throughout which your joints can move. The best way for you to maintain — or improve — the ROM of your joints is to perform specific flexibility movements to stretch the surrounding muscles. Flexibility movements are undoubtedly the simplest and most effortless physical activity that you can perform — the exertion level is quite low and relaxation is an absolute requirement. Nevertheless, many cross-training enthusiasts often overlook or underemphasize their flexibility training.

Increasing your flexibility serves several purposes. First of all, becoming more flexible generally makes you less susceptible to injury. Secondly, being more flexible enables you to exert your strength over a greater ROM. Finally, stretching your muscles is a way of relieving and/or reducing general muscle soreness that may result from unfamiliar activities or intense cross-training workouts.

FACTORS AFFECTING FLEXIBILITY

The most significant contributor to decreased flexibility seems to be a lack of physical activity. Obviously, you can avoid a loss of flexibility by simply participating in cross-training activities. However, there are many factors other than a sedentary lifestyle which also affect your ROM — some of which you have little or no control over.

There is a distinct relationship between your age and the degree of your flexibility. The greatest increase in flexibility usually occurs up to and between the ages of 7 and 12. During early adolescence, flexibility tends to level off and thereafter begins to decline with increasing age. Therefore, one of the goals of your flexibility program is to slow or perhaps reverse this decline.

To a degree, your flexibility is also related to your gender. Although some men are more flexible than some women, females are generally more flexible than males. Women retain this advantage throughout life.

In addition, it's important to understand that your flexibility is effected by several genetic or inherited characteristics such as the insertion points of your muscles and your ratio of muscle-to-fat (i.e., excessive body fat). Your ROM also has genetic structural limitations including your bones, tendons, ligaments and skin along with the extensibility of your muscles.

Previous injury to a muscle or connective tissue may also affect your ROM. Furthermore, immobilizing a joint during rehabilitation may cause your connective tissue to adapt to its shortest functional length thereby reducing the ROM of the joint.

Finally, your body temperature is another factor that influences joint flexibility. Muscles and connective tissue that are warmed-up will be more flexible and extensible than muscles and connective tissue that aren't warmed-up.

ASSESSING FLEXIBILITY

Because your ROM is affected by the aforementioned factors, it's difficult to assess flexibility in a fair manner. In addition, some measurements of flexibility can be misleading. A perfect example of this is the traditional sit-and-reach test in which a person sits down and reaches as far as possible. This test is often used to measure the flexibility of the lower back and the hamstrings. However, a sit-and-reach test does not take into consideration limb lengths. Everything else being equal, those with long arms and/or short legs have a distinct biomechanical advantage in a sit-and-reach test. These individuals may appear to be flexible but may actually be quite inflexible. Conversely, those with short arms and/or long legs have a distinct biomechanical disadvantage in a sit-and-reach test. These individuals may appear to be inflexible but may really be quite flexible. In the case of a sit-and-reach test, measuring the angle of flexion between the lumbar spine and the upper legs with a goniometer yields a more fair appraisal of flexibility. (A goniometer is a protractor-like instrument with two movable arms that enable you to measure joint angles.)

Lastly, it should be noted that your flexibility is joint-specific — a high degree of flexibility in one joint doesn't necessarily indicate high flexibility in other joints. Along these lines, it would not be uncommon for your flexibility to vary from one side of your body to the other.

In conclusion, the purpose of assessing flexibility should not be to compare your performance to that of someone else. Flexibility assessments are much more meaningful when your present flexibility is compared to your past flexibility.

"WARMING UP"

The research regarding the need for a "warm-up" seems to be inconclusive. Some studies have shown that a warm-up facilitates performance; other studies have shown that performances without a prior warm-up are no different than those with a warm-up. Nevertheless, a warm-up has both physiological and psychological importance.

For years, warming up was synonymous with stretching. However, warming up and stretching are two separate entities and must be treated as such. A warm-up is meant to prepare you for an upcoming session of cross training. On the other hand, the purpose of stretching is to induce a more long-term change in your ROM.

A warm-up should precede your flexibility training. Warm-up activities usually consist of low-intensity movements such as light jogging or calisthenics. Regardless of the warm-up activity, the idea is to systematically increase your body temperature and the blood flow to your muscles. Breaking a light sweat during the warm-up indicates that your body temperature has been raised sufficiently and that you are ready to begin stretching your muscles. As noted previously, muscles and connective tissue that are warmed-up have increased flexibility and extensibility. (In all likelihood, when the environmental temperature is high your body temperature is already elevated sufficiently to start stretching.)

Your biological tissue is most extensible at the end of your cross-training workout when your body temperature is elevated. Because of this, some authorities recommend that stretching should be performed after you have completed your workout. This may also reduce general muscle soreness after an intense cross-training activity.

By the way, there's no need for you to warm-up or stretch prior to strength training — provided that a relatively high number of repetitions are performed and the weight is lifted in a controlled manner. However, warming up prior to a cross-training activity involving rapid muscle contractions — such as sprinting — is advisable to reduce your risk of injury.

SEVEN STRETCHING STRATEGIES

Though the level of your flexibility may be limited by one or more of the factors previously mentioned, you can improve your ROM through an organized stretching program. Like all other forms of exercise, stretching movements have certain guidelines that must be followed in order to make the stretches safe and effective. Adopting these guidelines permits you to maintain or improve your current ROM. Additionally, you'll be less likely to get injured and will perform closer to your performance potential.

1. STRETCH under control without bouncing, bobbing or jerking movements. Bouncing during the stretch actually makes the movement more painful and increases your risk of muscle soreness and tissue damage.

2. INHALE and EXHALE normally during the stretch without holding your breath. Holding your breath elevates your blood pressure which disrupts your balance and breathing mechanisms.

3. STRETCH comfortably in a pain-free manner. Since pain is an indication that you are stretching at or near your structural limits, you should only stretch to a point of mild discomfort.

4. RELAX during the stretch. Relaxing mentally and physically allows you to stretch your muscles throughout a greater ROM.

5. HOLD the stretched position for 30 - 60 seconds. Gradually stretching your muscles to a point of mild discomfort, holding that position and then gradually returning them to their pre-stretched state enables you to stretch farther with little risk of pain or injury.

6. ATTEMPT to stretch a little bit farther than the last time. Progressively increasing your ROM — and the time that each stretch is held — improves your flexibility.

7. PERFORM flexibility movements on a regular basis. You should stretch at least once a day, especially before a practice, game, cross-training session or any other activity that involves explosive, ballistic movements.

FLEXIBILITY EXERCISES

Although your body has roughly 200 joints, it isn't necessary to perform a flexibility movement for each one. Your joints range from those that are relatively immovable (e.g., the sutures of your skull) to those that are freely movable (e.g., your hips and your elbows). You can stretch the muscles of your major joints in a comprehensive manner by performing the 14 flexibility movements which are described on the following pages. Each movement lists the muscle(s) stretched, a brief description for each movement and performance points on making the exercise safer and more effective. (For help in identifying the muscles, an anatomy chart is shown in Chapter 2.) The stretches described in this chapter are the neck forward, neck backward, lateral neck, scratch back, handcuff, standing calf, tibia stretch, sit-and-reach, V-sit, lateral reach, butterfly, spinal twist, quad stretch and knee pull. There are many variations of these stretches that involve the same muscle groups. As such, your stretching program can be individualized to meet your personal preferences. *(All photos in this section taken by Matt Brzycki)*

NECK FORWARD

Muscles stretched: neck extensors, trapezius

Description: Interlock your fingers behind your head and slowly pull your chin to your chest.

Performance Points:

1. Be especially careful when performing this stretch since your cervical area is involved.

2. This movement may also be performed sitting.

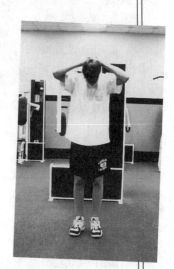

NECK BACKWARD

Muscles stretched: sternocleidomastoideus

Description: Place your hands underneath your chin and slowly push your head backward.

Performance Points:

1. Be especially careful when performing this stretch since your cervical area is involved.

2. This movement may also be performed sitting.

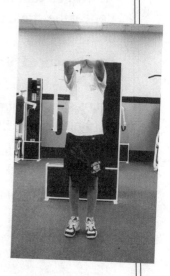

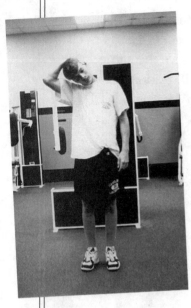

LATERAL NECK

Muscles stretched: sternocleidomastoideus (one side)

Description: Place your right hand on the left side of your head and slowly pull your head to your right shoulder. Repeat the stretch for the right side of your neck.

Performance Points:

1. Be especially careful when performing this stretch since your cervical area is involved.

2. This movement may also be performed sitting.

SCRATCH BACK

Muscles stretched: upper back (lats), triceps, obliques

Description: Place your left hand on the upper part of your back (behind your head), grab your left elbow with your right hand and slowly pull your upper torso to the right. Repeat the stretch for the right side of your body.

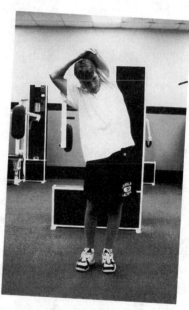

Performance Points:

1. For this stretch to be most effective, your hips should not move and your feet should remain flat on the ground.

2. You should try to gradually reach farther down your back during the stretch.

3. This movement may also be performed sitting.

4. This movement may be contraindicated for individuals with shoulder impingement syndrome.

HANDCUFF

Muscles stretched: chest, anterior deltoid, biceps

Description: Place your hands behind your back, interlock your fingers and slowly lift your hands up as high as possible.

Performance Points:

1. A partner may assist you in obtaining a greater stretch by carefully lifting up your hands as you perform the stretch.

2. This movement may also be performed sitting.

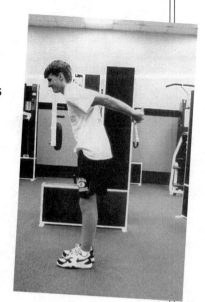

STANDING CALF

Muscle stretched: calves, iliopsoas

Description: While standing upright, step forward with your right foot. Bend your right leg at the knee but keep your left leg straight and your left foot flat on the ground. Repeat the stretch for your right leg.

Performance Points:

1. For this stretch to be most effective, the heel of your back foot should remain flat on the ground and both of your feet should be pointed forward.

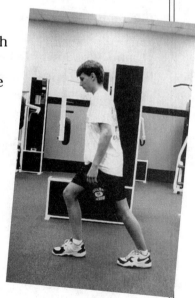

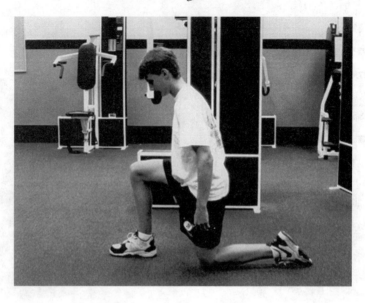

TIBIA STRETCH

Muscle stretched: dorsi flexors

Description: Kneel down on your left knee so that your upper leg is perpendicular to the ground while your lower leg and the top part of your foot is flat on the ground. Position your right leg so that your upper leg is parallel to the ground, your lower leg is perpendicular to the ground and your foot is flat on the ground. Repeat the stretch for your right dorsi flexors.

Performance Points:

1. For this stretch to be most effective, the top part of the foot being stretched should be flat on the ground.

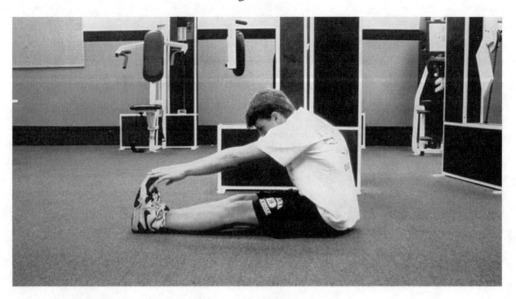

SIT-AND-REACH

Muscles stretched: buttocks, hamstrings, calves, upper back (lats), lower back

Description: Straighten your legs, put them together and point your toes upward. Slowly reach forward as far as possible without bending your legs.

Performance Points:

1. For this stretch to be most effective, your legs should remain straight and your toes should be pointed upward.

2. You can progressively stretch farther by reaching for your ankles, your toes and finally your instep.

3. A partner may assist you in obtaining a greater stretch by carefully pushing on your upper back as you perform the stretch.

4. This movement may also be performed standing (with your legs straight and your arms hanging straight down).

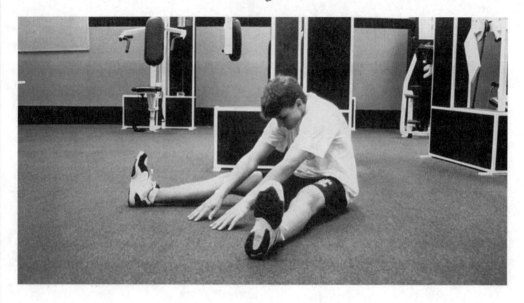

V-SIT

Muscles stretched: buttocks, hip adductors (inner thigh), hamstrings, calves, upper back (lats), lower back

Description: Straighten your legs, spread them apart as far as possible and point your toes upward. Slowly reach forward as far as possible without bending your legs.

Performance Points:

1. For this stretch to be most effective, your legs should remain straight and your toes should be pointed upward.

2. You can progressively stretch farther by "walking" your fingers forward.

3. A partner may assist you in obtaining a greater stretch by carefully pushing on your upper back as you perform the stretch.

4. This movement may also be performed standing (with your legs spread apart and your arms hanging straight down).

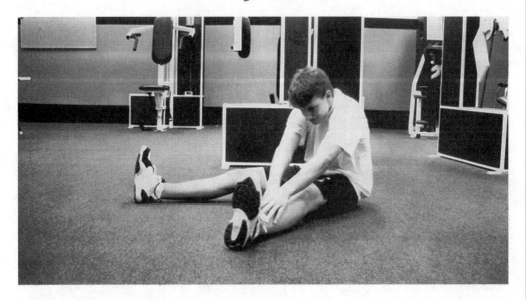

LATERAL REACH

Muscles stretched: buttocks, hip adductors (inner thigh), hamstrings, calves, upper back (lats), obliques, lower back

Description: Straighten your legs, spread them apart as far as possible and point your toes upward. Slowly reach down your left leg as far as possible without bending your legs. Repeat the stretch for the right side of your body.

Performance Points:

1. For this stretch to be most effective, your legs should remain straight and your toes should be pointed upward.

2. You can progressively stretch farther by "walking" your fingers forward.

3. A partner may assist you in obtaining a greater stretch by carefully pushing on your upper back as you perform the stretch.

4. This movement may also be performed standing (with your legs spread apart and your arms reaching down your leg).

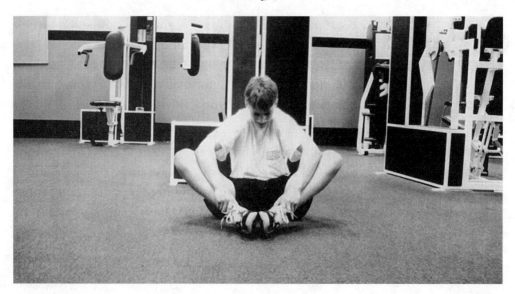

BUTTERFLY

Muscles stretched: hip adductors (inner thigh), lower back

Description: Place the soles of your feet together, draw your heels as close to your buttocks as possible and place your elbows on the insides of your knees. Bend your torso forward while slowly pushing down with your elbows against your knees.

Performance Points:

1.A partner may assist you in obtaining a greater stretch by carefully pushing on the insides of your knees as you perform the stretch.

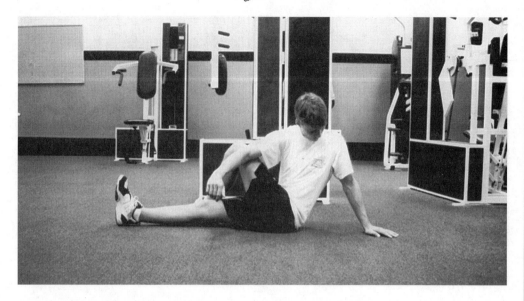

SPINAL TWIST

Muscles stretched: hip abductors (gluteus medius), obliques, lower back

Description: Keep your right leg straight, place your left foot on the outside of your right knee, place your right elbow against the outside of your left knee and look to your left as far as possible. Repeat the stretch for the other side of your body.

Performance Points:

1. This exercise may also be performed laying supine (by keeping your shoulders flat on the ground and crossing one leg over your body).

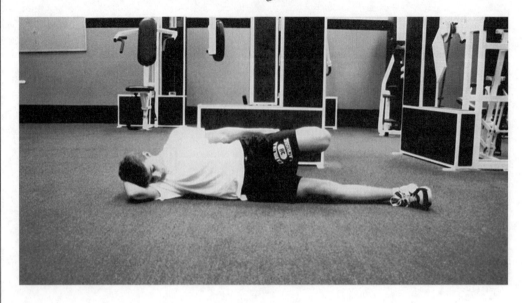

QUAD STRETCH

Muscles stretched: quadriceps, iliopsoas, abdominals

Description: Lay on your right side, grab your left instep with your left hand and pull your heel toward your buttocks. Repeat the stretch for the right side of your body.

Performance Points:

1. This movement may also be performed laying prone.

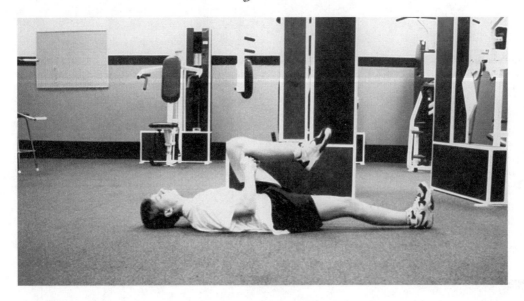

KNEE PULL

Muscles stretched: buttocks, hamstrings, lower back

Description: Lay supine on the ground with your legs extended. Grasp your left leg behind your knee and pull it toward your chest. Keep your right leg straight and your toes pointed upward. Repeat the stretch for the right side of your body.

Performance Points:

1. Using your arms to pull your leg toward your chest will permit a better stretch.

⑼ Nutrition for Successful Cross Training

Nutrition is the process by which you select, consume, digest, absorb and utilize food. Unfortunately, this aspect of overall fitness is often overlooked and seldom addressed. Proper nutrition plays a critical role in your capacity to perform at optimal levels and to expedite your recovery. Truly, your ability to fully recuperate after an exhaustive activity directly effects your future performance and subsequent intensity in your cross training. Your nutritional habits are also a factor in the development of your muscular size and strength.

Your nutritional "skills" can be improved by knowing the desirable food sources, the recommended intakes of those food sources and the physiological contributions of the various nutrients. It's also meaningful to examine your caloric "needs" along with the principles and procedures for weight management (i.e., gaining, losing or maintaining weight). A knowledge of what foods to eat before and after vigorous activity is helpful in maximizing performance. Finally, it's important to understand the potential dangers of excessive nutritional supplementation.

THE NUTRIENTS

Everything that you do requires energy. Energy is measured in calories and is obtained through the foods — or nutrients — that you eat. Essentially, the foods that you consume serve as a fuel for your body. Food is also necessary for the growth, maintenance and repair of your body tissue such as muscle and bone.

Foods are composed of six nutrients: carbohydrates, proteins, fats, water, vitamins and minerals. These six main constituents of food are divided into the macronutrients and the micronutrients. In order to be considered "nutritious," your food intake must contain the recommended percentages of the macronutrients as well as appropriate levels of the micronutrients. No single foodstuff satisfies this requirement. As such, variety is the key to a well-balanced diet.

The Macronutrients

As the name implies, macronutrients are needed in relatively large amounts. Three macronutrients — carbohydrates, proteins and fats — provide you with a supply of energy. Although it has no calories, water is also considered a macronutrient because it's needed in considerable quantities.

Carbohydrates. The primary job of carbohydrates — or "carbs" — is to supply you with energy, especially during intense activity. Your body breaks down carbohydrates into glucose or "blood sugar." Glucose can be used as an immediate form of energy during exercise or stored as glycogen in your liver and muscles for future use. Highly conditioned muscles can stockpile more glycogen than poorly conditioned muscles. When glycogen stores are depleted, a person feels overwhelmingly exhausted. For this reason, greater glycogen stores can provide you with a physiological advantage. Therefore, your diet should be carbohydrate-based. In fact, at least 65 percent of your daily food intake should be in the form of carbohydrates.

Carbohydrates are found in sugars (such as table sugar and honey), starches (like the starch in bread) and fibers. Carbohydrate-rich foods include potatoes, cereals, pancakes, breads, spaghetti, macaroni, rice, grains, fruits and vegetables.

Proteins. Protein is necessary for the repair, maintenance and growth of your biological tissue — particularly muscle tissue. In addition, protein regulates your water balance and transports other nutrients. Protein can also be used as an energy source in the event that adequate carbohydrates aren't available. Good sources of protein are beef, pork, fish, poultry, eggs, liver, dry beans and dairy products.

When proteins are ingested as foods, they are broken down into their basic "building blocks": amino acids. Of the 22 known amino acids, your body can manufacture 13 of them. The other 9, however, must be provided in your diet and are termed "essential amino acids." When a food contains all of the essential amino acids, it is called a "complete protein." All animal proteins — with the exception of gelatin — are complete proteins. The protein found in vegetables and other sources is "incomplete protein" because it doesn't include all of the essential amino acids. Approximately 15 percent of your daily food consumption should be protein.

Fats. It's hard to believe, but fats are essential to a balanced diet. First of all, fats serve as a major source of energy during activities of low intensity such as sleeping, reading and walking. This nutrient also helps in the transportation and the absorption of certain vitamins. Lastly, fats add considerable flavor to foods. This makes food more appetizing — and also explains why fats are craved so much.

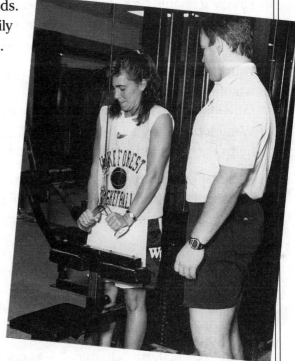

Foods high in fat are butter, cheese, margarine, meat, nuts, milk products and cooking oils. Animal fats — such as butter, lard and the fat in meats — are usually dubbed "saturated" and contribute to heart disease; vegetable fats — such as corn oil and peanut oil — are generally "unsaturated" and less harmful. (At room temperature, saturated fats tend to be solid and unsaturated fats are usually liquid.)

There's really no need for you to add extra "fatty" food to your diet in order to get adequate fat. If anything, the average American consumes far too much fat. The fact is that fats often accompany carbohydrate and protein choices. In addition, foods are frequently prepared in such a way that the fat content is elevated. For example, a potato is generally an excellent source of carbohydrates. However, preparing a potato as french fries increases the number of fat calories much more than preparing it baked. At most, 20 percent of your daily food intake should be composed of fats. Keep in mind that this allotment of fat — as well as that of carbohydrates and proteins — is meant to be distributed over the course of the day. So, there's nothing wrong with eating a food that exceeds 20-percent fat as long as this particular choice is balanced out by other foods consumed throughout the day.

Above: The primary job of carbohydrates — or "carbs" — is to supply you with energy, especially during intense activity. (Photo provided by Wake Forest University)

Finally, it should be noted that carbohydrates and proteins are converted into fat if not utilized by your body. Any fats that aren't used as energy are also stored as fats.

Water. Although it doesn't have any calories or provide you with energy, water is sometimes classified as a macronutrient because it's needed in rather large quantities. In fact, almost two thirds of your bodyweight is water. Water lubricates your joints and regulates your body temperature. Water also helps carry nutrients to your cells and waste products away from your cells.

The best sources of water are milk, fruit juices, soup and, of course, water. You should consume about 16 ounces of water for every pound of weight that you lose during your cross-training activities.

The Micronutrients

Vitamins and minerals are classified as micronutrients because they are needed in rather small amounts. Neither of these nutrients supplies you with any calories or energy. However, vitamins and minerals have many other important functions.

Vitamins. The term "vitamine" was coined by the Polish chemist Casimir Funk in 1912. Vitamins are potent compounds that are required in very small quantities. As noted earlier, these substances are not a source of energy but perform many different roles. For instance, vitamin A helps maintain your vision at night, vitamin C is necessary for your wounds to heal, vitamin D is vital for strong bones and teeth, vitamin E protects and maintains your cellular membranes and vitamin K is essential for blood clotting. Vitamins occur in a wide variety of foods, especially in fruits and vegetables. You can obtain an adequate intake of vitamins from a balanced diet that contains a variety of foods.

Vitamins can be classified as either fat-soluble or water-soluble. The four fat-soluble vitamins — vitamins A, D, E and K — require proper amounts of fat to be present before transportation and absorption can take place. Excessive amounts of fat-soluble vitamins are stored in your body. The eight B vitamins (thiamine, riboflavin, niacin, pantothenic acid, pyridoxine, cobalamin, biotin and folic acid) and vitamin C are considered water-soluble vitamins be-cause they are found in foods that have a naturally high content of water. There is minimal storage of water-soluble vitamins in your body — excess amounts are generally excreted in your urine.

Minerals. Minerals are found in tiny amounts in foods. Like vitamins, nearly all the minerals that you need can be obtained with an ordinary intake of foods.

Calcium, phosphorus, magnesium, potassium, iron and zinc are among the 21 essential minerals that must be provided by your food intake. Minerals have many vital purposes such as building strong bones and teeth, helping your muscles function properly and even enabling your heart to beat.

DAILY SERVINGS

Indulging in an assortment of foods ensures that you've obtained a sufficient amount of each type of macronutrient along with a healthy quantity of essential vitamins and minerals. According to the U. S. Department of Agriculture, a variety of daily foods would include choices from these six food groups: 6 - 11 servings from the Bread, Cereal, Rice and Pasta Group; 3 - 5 servings from the Vegetable Group; 2 - 4 servings from the Fruit Group; 2 - 3 servings from the Milk, Yogurt and Cheese Group; 2 - 3 servings from the Meat, Poultry, Fish, Dry Beans, Eggs and Nuts Group; and a conservative amount from the Fats, Oils and Sweets Group.

RECOMMENDED DIETARY ALLOWANCES

The Recommended Dietary Allowances (RDAs) are established by the National Research Council of the National Academy of Sciences. The RDAs are set by first determining the "floor" below which deficiency occurs and then by determining the "ceiling" above which harm occurs. A margin of safety is included in the RDAs to meet the needs of nearly all healthy people. In fact, the RDAs are designed to cover 97.5 percent of the population. In other words, the RDAs exceed what most people require in order to meet the needs of individuals with the highest requirements. The RDAs do not represent minimum requirements and any failure to consume the recommended amounts doesn't necessarily indicate you have a dietary deficiency.

CALORIC CONTRIBUTIONS

It's necessary to understand that carbohydrates, proteins and fats provide different amounts of calories. Carbohydrates and proteins yield 4 calories per gram (cal/g). Fats are the most concentrated form of energy, containing 9 cal/g. (Alcohol provides 7 cal/g.) With this information, you can determine the caloric contributions for each of the energy-providing macronutrients in any food — provided that you know how many grams of each macronutrient are in a serving. For example, suppose a nutrition label notes that one serving of a certain food has 16 grams of carbohydrate, 2 grams of protein and 8 grams of fat. To find the number of calories that are supplied by each macronutrient, simply multiply its number of grams per serving by its corresponding energy yield. In this example, each serving of the food has 64 calories from carbohydrates [16 g x 4 cal/g], 8 calories from protein [2 g x 4

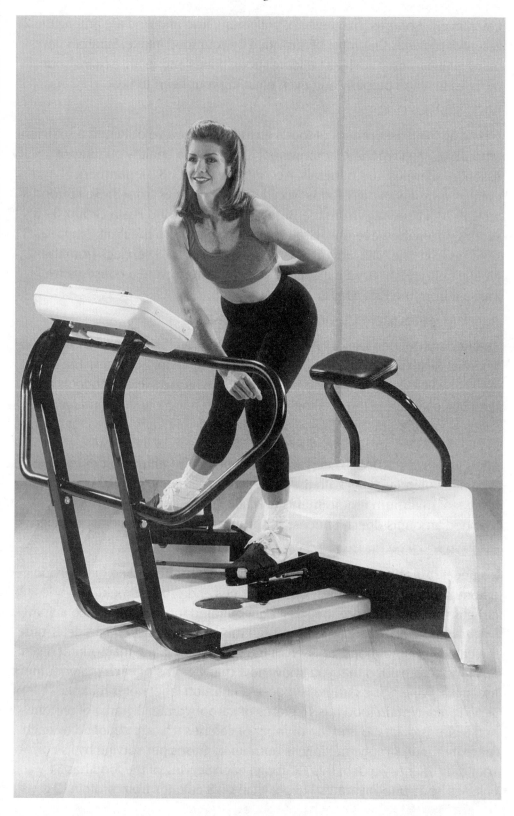

cal/g] and 72 calories from fat [8 g x 9 cal/g]. Therefore, this food has a total of 144 calories per serving. Note that even though this particular food has twice as many grams of carbohydrates as fats (16 compared to 8), exactly 50 percent of the calories (72 of the 144) are furnished by fats. Incidentally, this food is actually typical of a popular snack food: potato chips.

Knowing the different caloric contributions of the macronutrients is also helpful in understanding food labels that may contain misleading information about fat content. A food label proclaiming a product as being "95-percent fat-free" means that it's 95-percent fat-free by weight . . . not by calories. Placing 5 grams of fat into 95 grams of water forms a product that, by weight, is 95-percent fat-free. Since water has no calories, however, this particular "95-percent fat-free" product would actually be 100-percent fat in terms of calories.

ESTIMATING YOUR CALORIC "BUDGET"

Your need for calories — or energy — is determined by several factors including your age, gender, body composition, metabolic rate and activity level. Your caloric requirements during a resting state can be determined precisely by both direct and indirect calorimetry. Direct calorimetry measures the heat produced by the body in a small, insulated chamber; indirect calorimetry calculates the heat given off by the body based upon the amounts of oxygen consumed and carbon dioxide produced. These methods can be costly and impractical for most people. For a quick and reasonably accurate estimate of your daily caloric needs, the U. S. Department of Agriculture suggests multiplying your bodyweight by a number that is determined by your level of activity. Essentially, this number represents your energy requirements in calories per pound of bodyweight (cal/lb). For females, the values are 14 if the woman is sedentary, 18 if she is moderately active and 22 if she is very active; for males, the factors are 16, 21 and 26, respectively. As an example, a 200-pound male who is very active requires about 5,200 calories per day (cal/day) to meet his energy needs [200 lb x 26 cal/lb].

Once you've estimated your caloric "budget," your next step is to determine how many of these calories should come from carbohydrates, proteins and fats. Using the previous example, someone who requires about 5,200 cal/day should consume about 845 grams of carbohydrates [5,200 cal/day times .65 divided by 4 cal/g], 195 grams of proteins [5,200 cal/day times .15 divided by

---

Left: Your need for calories — or energy — is determined by several factors including your age, gender, body composition, metabolic rate and activity level. (Photo provided by Nautilus International)

4 cal/g] and 116 grams of fat [5,200 cal/day times .20 divided by 9 cal/g]. It should be noted that these numbers are based upon a diet that consists of 65-percent carbohydrates, 15-percent proteins and 20-percent fats.

WEIGHT MANAGEMENT

Gaining, losing or maintaining bodyweight is simply a matter of arithmetic and can be likened to bank transactions. If you deposit (consume) more calories than you withdraw (expend), you've produced a "caloric profit" and gain weight; if you withdraw (expend) more calories than you deposit (consume), you've established a "caloric deficit" and lose weight; and lastly, if you deposit (consume) the same amount of calories that you withdraw (expend), a "caloric balance" is produced and your bodyweight doesn't change. However, a closer inspection of gaining and losing weight is necessary.

Gaining Weight

 The potential to gain weight is determined by several factors, the most important of which is an individual's genetic make-up. A person whose ancestors have ectomorphic tendencies (i.e., long limbs and slender builds) has the genetic destiny for a very similar physique. This doesn't mean that an ectomorphic person cannot gain weight. However, someone who has a high degree of ectomorphy will have a difficult time increasing bodyweight significantly.

The principal goal in gaining weight is to increase lean body mass. One pound of muscle has about 2,500 calories. Therefore, if someone consumes 250 cal/day above the caloric budget (i.e., a 250-calorie "profit"), it will take 10 days to add one pound of lean, fat-free weight [2,500 cal divided by 250 cal/day equals 10 days]. So, if the previously mentioned 200-pound individual requires 5,200 cal/day to maintain his bodyweight, he must consume 5,450 cal/day (i.e., 250 calories above his need) to gain one pound of fat-free weight in 10 days. This estimate must be recalculated on a regular basis to account for the greater bodyweight. After increasing his bodyweight to 201 pounds, he'll now require 5,226 cal/day to meet his energy needs [201 lb x 26 cal/lb]. In order to gain another pound in 10 days, he must increase his caloric consumption to 5,476 cal/day (i.e., 250 calories above his need).

It should be noted that the daily caloric profit should not be more than about 1,000 - 1,500 calories above the normal daily caloric intake. If the weight gain is more than about two pounds per week, it's likely that some excess calories will be stored in the form of fat. However, if the weight gain is less than about two pounds per week and is the result of a demanding strength-training program in conjunction with a well-balanced nutritional intake, then it will probably be in the form of increased muscle tissue.

Proper weight gain relies upon total nutritional dedication for 7 days a week. Additional calories must be consumed daily on a regular basis until the desired weight gain is achieved. The body absorbs food best when it is divided into several regular-sized meals intermingled with a few snacks. One or two large meals aren't absorbed by the body as well — most of these calories are simply jammed through the digestive system. In fact, if a large number of calories is consumed at one time, some calories will be diverted to fat deposits because of the sudden demand on the metabolic pathways. (This has been referred to as "nutrient overload.")

Losing Weight

The numbers on a height-weight chart or a bathroom scale are a poor indicator of whether or not a person should lose weight. The need for weight loss should be determined by body composition rather than bodyweight — especially in the case of an athlete. In general, athletes tend to be larger and more muscular than the rest of the population. As an example, suppose two people are 6 feet tall and weigh 220 pounds. If you consider their height and weight without regard for their body composition, you might conclude that they're both overweight. However, what if one person had 20-percent body fat and the other had 10-percent body fat? If this was the case, then only one person needed to lose weight — the one with the higher percentage of body fat. As such, determining the need to lose weight should be based upon body composition.

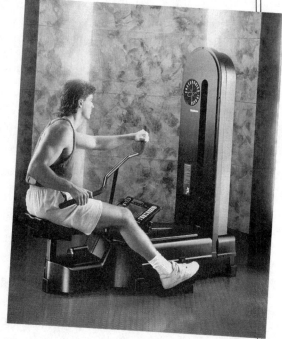

Body fat can be measured in a variety of ways, although using skinfold calipers is generally considered to be the most practical method of assessment. Men and women should maintain a body fat of about 12 - 18 per-

Left: Proper weight loss should be a combination of reducing the caloric intake and increasing the energy expenditure — such as through additional cross-training activities. (Photo by StairMaster Sports/Medical Products, Inc.)

cent and 16 - 25 percent, respectively. Normal body fats for athletes are lower than the average population, ranging from about 5 - 13 percent for males and 12 - 22 percent for females. Body fats in excess of 25 percent in males and 32 percent in females are considered unhealthy.

The primary goal of a weight-loss program is to decrease body fat. One pound of fat has about 3,500 calories. As such, if someone expends 250 cal/day below the caloric budget (i.e., a 250-calorie "deficit"), it will take 14 days to lose one pound of fat [3,500 cal divided by 250 cal/day equals 14 days]. In this instance, if the 200-pound individual in the ongoing example needs 5,200 cal/day to maintain his bodyweight, he must consume 4,950 cal/day (i.e., 250 calories below his need) to lose one pound of fat in 14 days. This estimate must be recalculated on a regular basis to account for the lower bodyweight. After decreasing his bodyweight to 199 pounds, he'll now require 5,174 cal/day to meet his energy needs [199 lb x 26 cal/lb]. In order to lose another pound in 14 days, he must decrease his caloric consumption to 4,924 cal/day (i.e., 250 calories below his need).

A caloric deficit can be achieved by reducing the caloric intake, increasing the energy expenditure (such as through additional aerobic cross training) or a combination of the two. In fact, proper weight loss should be a blend of dieting and exercise. It should be noted that the daily caloric deficit should not be more than about 1,000 - 1,500 calories below the normal daily caloric intake. If the weight loss is more than about two pounds per week, it's likely that some of this weight reduction will be the result of decreased muscle tissue and/or water rather than body fat.

Weight loss must be a carefully planned activity. Skipping meals — or all-out starvation — isn't a desirable method of weight loss, since fuel is still needed for an active lifestyle. Oddly enough, losing weight should be done in a fashion similar to gaining weight. Frequent — but smaller — meals spread out over the course of the day suppresses the appetite. Drinking plenty of water before, during and after meals creates a feeling of fullness without providing any calories.

THE PRE-ACTIVITY MEAL

A meal consumed prior to a competition or a cross-training activity should accomplish several things such as removing your hunger pangs, fueling your body for the upcoming activity and settling you psychologically. No foods consumed several hours before a contest or an activity lead directly to a greater or improved performance. However, there are certain foods that you should avoid prior to a competition or activity. For example, fats and meats are digested slowly. This means that the traditional steak dinner might actually be the worst possible meal for you to eat before a competition. Other foods to omit include those that are greasy, highly seasoned and flatulent (gas-forming), along with any specific foods that you may personally find distressful to your digestive system. If anything, the choices for your pre-activity meal should be almost bland, yet appetizing enough so that you want to eat it.

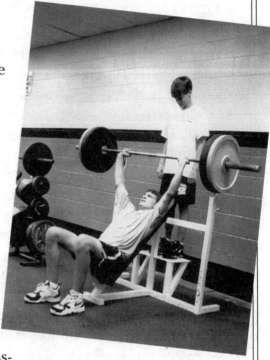

You should also avoid consuming large amounts of sugar or sweets — such as candy or soda — less than one hour before a competition or a cross-training activity. Sugar consumption causes a sharp increase in your blood glucose levels. In response, your body increases its blood insulin levels to maintain a stable internal environment. As a result of this chemical balancing, your blood glucose is sharply reduced leading to hypoglycemia — or 'low blood sugar" — which decreases the availability of blood glucose as a fuel and causes you to feel severely fatigued.

The best foods that you can consume prior to a competition or a cross-training activity are carbohydrates. Carbohydrates are easily digested and help maintain your blood glucose levels within a desirable range. Water is perhaps the best liquid for you to drink before competing or exercising. Your fluid intake should be enough to guarantee optimal hydration during the activity.

The timing of your pre-activity meal is also crucial. To ensure that the digestive process doesn't impair your performance, you shouldn't eat your pre-activity meal less than three hours before a competition or an activity. In short, your pre-activity meal should include foods that are familiar and well-tolerated — preferably carbohydrates.

Right: The protein intakes of highly active individuals are typically well above the RDA for protein and adequately cover any increased need that may be related to strength training or other cross-training activities. (Photo by Matt Brzycki)

RECOVERY FOODS/FLUIDS

After intense activity or competition, proper nutrition accelerates your recovery and better prepares you for your next physical endeavor. To replenish your depleted glycogen stores and to expedite the recovery process, you should consume foods that are high in carbohydrates as soon as possible following exhaustive activity. Because your appetite is suppressed immediately after intense efforts, it may be more practical for you to consume a high-carbohydrate beverage rather than solid food or a meal. (A cold beverage also helps cool off your body.) Several commercial sports drinks are high in carbohydrates, but you should read the label to be sure of its exact content. According to nutritionist Nancy Clark, a person should ingest 0.5 grams of carbohydrates per pound of bodyweight (g/lb) within two hours of completing an intense competition or activity. This should be repeated again within the next two hours. For instance, a person weighing 200 pounds needs to consume about 100 grams of carbohydrates (or 400 carbohydrate calories) within two hours after intense physical activity and another 100 grams of carbohydrates during the next two hours [0.5 g/lb x 200 lb = 100 g].

NUTRITIONAL SUPPLEMENTS

Skillful promoters of nutritional supplements have bestowed protein, amino acids, vitamins, minerals, herbs and other substances with almost supernatural powers having the ability to do practically everything imaginable. Consumers are frequently tempted, teased and seduced by brilliant promises of "losing flab," "gaining muscle" and "getting fit". Because of this, many people don't give a second thought to spending huge sums of their money on a never-ending parade of nutritional "supplements" that claim to improve overall health, physical appearance and athletic performance.

Unfortunately, Americans spend more than 25 billion dollars each year on health quackery — about half of which goes for health-food pills, powders and potions. The fact of the matter is that most of the claims concerning nutritional supplements are purely speculative and anecdotal with little or no scientific or medical basis.

Protein and Amino Acids

The need for a high intake of dietary protein and/or amino acid supplements by those who engage in rigorous physical activity has been drastically exaggerated and overrated by health-food manufacturers and promoters. The truth is, there are no significant nutritional benefits obtained from the intake of additional dietary protein or amino acid supplements by those consuming adequate diets. Protein is critical to daily existence, but it won't give you any superhuman powers. There is no consistent scientific evidence that indicates a high protein intake or amino acid supplementation improves performance or increases muscle mass. Furthermore, high protein intakes — in excess of 2 - 3 times the RDA — have not been shown to enhance physical endurance or muscular strength. An overwhelming number of researchers, scientists, strength and fitness practitioners, scientific nutritionists, registered dietitians and physicians have noted that a high intake of protein or amino acid supplementation is unnecessary for individuals who consume a well-balanced diet.

Protein needs. Most Americans — including those at the bottom of the socioeconomic scale — receive more than enough protein. It has been suggested, however, that active individuals require greater amounts of dietary protein. Studies have shown that the protein needs of individuals involved in intense strength-training programs may be higher than those of sedentary individuals. Nevertheless, the protein intakes of highly active individuals are typically well above the RDA for protein and adequately cover any increased need that may be related to strength training or other cross-training activities. Some research even suggests that an improved metabolic efficiency allows exercisers to meet enhanced demands for protein without requiring an increased protein intake.

Individuals who consume adequate calories generally obtain sufficient protein. Recall that your caloric requirements are determined by several factors including your body composition and activity level. Larger, more active individuals require and consume more calories than the average person. With these additional calories come additional protein. In other words, the increased protein need is met by increased caloric intake.

The RDA for protein is 0.8 grams per kilogram of bodyweight per day (g/kg/ day) for adults. Assuming sufficient caloric intake, 1.2 - 2.0 g/kg/day (about 150 - 250 percent of the RDA for adults) is present in any mixed diet that contains 12 - 15 percent of its calories as protein. Recall the 200-pound individual in the ongoing example who must consume 5,200 cal/day to maintain his bodyweight. If 15 percent of these calories came from protein, he would be receiving 780 calories from protein or 195 grams [780 cal divided by 4 cal/g equals 195 g]. Based upon the RDA of 0.8 g/kg/day, this individual would be consuming enough protein to meet the daily needs of a 536-pound man [195 g/day divided by 0.8g/kg/day times 2.2 lb/kg equals 536.25 lb]. This amount of protein is actually about 2.15 g/kg/day — or about

2.5 times the RDA — without the person making any effort to consume extra dietary protein or using amino acid supplements. Even if the requirement for active individuals may be greater, it's likely that they are already consuming enough protein to ensure proper levels of consumption. If anything, an inadequate intake of carbohydrates is more often a problem than an inadequate intake of protein.

Clearly, there is no need for a high protein intake or for amino acid supplements if you consume enough calories. If you are concerned that you're not getting enough protein in your diet, you can obtain sufficient protein by simply consuming more foods that are high in protein.

Excessive protein intake. There are numerous unwanted side effects related to an excessive intake of protein — several of which may be physically detrimental. A high protein intake in excess of the needs for building body tissue and essential body compounds is either stored as fat or excreted in the urine. Excreting excessive protein in the urine places a heavy burden on the liver and kidneys and may damage those organs. An excessive intake of protein also increases the risk of dehydration as a result of the extra water that is required to rid the body of the by-products of protein metabolism. Dehydration increases the risk of developing a heat-related disorder such as heat exhaustion, heat stroke or heat cramps. (Heat disorders are detailed in Chapter 12.) Other side effects from a high protein intake include an excessive loss of calcium in the urine, an increased risk of renal disease, diarrhea, cramping, gout and gastrointestinal upset.

The hype-inspired use of amino acid supplements by large numbers of individuals has generated considerable concern for consumer safety. In 1992, the Federation of American Societies for Experimental Biology reviewed the scientific literature on the safety of amino acids and reported that there is insufficient scientific evidence to establish safe levels of intake of the amino acid supplements on the market. Additionally, the American Council of Science and Health recommends, "Unless you are participating in a scientific study conducted by reputable researchers, you should not take amino acid supplements since they have not been proven safe."

Vitamins and Minerals

Vitamins and minerals make up more than 80 percent of the sales in the multi-billion dollar dietary supplement market. Vitamins and minerals — like proteins and amino acids — have also been thought to have magical powers. The belief is that if the RDA is good, then more must be better. It's true that a deficiency of vitamins and minerals can make you unhealthy, but consuming more than you need won't necessarily make you any healthier. Your liver is a storehouse for vitamins and minerals. This organ can quickly compensate for a temporary dietary shortfall by releasing its stored nutrients as needed and then replenishing its reservoirs when the opportunity arises. Despite this, millions of Americans believe that their foods do not supply adequate vitamins and minerals and, therefore, they take nutritional supplements — often in potentially dangerous megadoses which sometimes result in actual harm.

Like protein and amino acid supplementation, there is little evidence to suggest that vitamin and mineral supplementation in excess of the RDA is needed by those who consume a well-balanced diet. A 1988 study concluded "multivitamin and mineral supplementation was without any measurable ergogenic effect" and that "supplementation is unnecessary in athletes ingesting a normal diet." There is simply no evidence that increased vitamin consumption improves performance. Moreover, there doesn't appear to be an increased demand for most vitamins and minerals during periods of increased physical activity. Recall that active individuals require and consume more calories than the average person. With these additional calories come additional vitamins and minerals.

As a result of the increased knowledge and the availability of a variety of foods rich in vitamins and minerals, deficiency diseases are rare in the United States and other industrialized nations. There is no risk of a vitamin and mineral deficiency due to the volume of food consumed — even a marginal diet provides adequate vitamins and minerals. If a normal intake of vitamins and minerals was insufficient, there would be an abundance of deficiency diseases such as beriberi (thiamin), cheilosis (riboflavin), pellegra (niacin), scurvy (vitamin C), rickets (vitamin D) and kwashiorkor (magnesium and protein). In fact, the only commonly documented deficiency in the United States is iron. Other than iron deficiency, physicians rarely encounter any nutrient-deficiency disease except in chronic alcoholics or people with an underlying illness that interferes with their food intake or metabolism.

Whenever possible, it's better to get vitamins from foods rather than pills because the high concentration of a vitamin or a mineral in pill form may interfere with the absorption of some other nutrients. However, vitamin and mineral supplements may be necessary for improving the nutrient intake of those who consume inadequate diets. For example, a multi-vitamin and mineral supplement may be warranted for vegetarians, some infants and pregnant or lactating females. Supplementation may also be appropriate for someone consuming a low number of calories such as those restricting their caloric intake to reach a certain weight class to compete in boxing, wrestling or judo. Supplements containing more than 150 percent of the RDA are for disease treatment and should never be purchased unless a competent health professional has diagnosed a need for them. Professional advice concerning nutritional supplementation should be sought from a registered dietitian (R.D.) or a nutritionist. With few exceptions, vitamin and mineral supplementation is a waste of money.

Excessive vitamin intake. When sold at reasonable potencies — as most of them are — vitamins (and minerals) pose no health or safety problems. However, megadoses of vitamins (i.e., any dose greater than 10 times the RDA) carry a risk of toxicity which can create adverse side effects and may lead to serious medical complications. The American Dietetic Association — the largest and best established organization devoted to both practice and research in nutrition — reports that vitamins (and minerals) pose a risk of toxicity. When taken in megadose amounts, the vitamins that are in excess of those needed to saturate the enzyme systems function as free-floating drugs instead of receptor-bound nutrients. Like all drugs, high doses of vitamins (and minerals) have the potential for adverse side effects. Though excess amounts of water-soluble vitamins are mainly excreted in the urine, they still may have toxic effects. Of greatest concern is excessive intake of the fat-soluble vitamins, particularly vitamins A and D which can be extremely toxic and may have adverse side effects.

Permanent effects of vitamin A toxicity are rare. However, consuming large doses of vitamin A can be dangerous and even lethal. Excessive doses of vitamin A can result in the following side effects: nausea, drowsiness, diarrhea, decalcification of the bones (resulting in fragile bones), an increased susceptibility to disease, muscle and joint soreness, vomiting, cessation of menstruation (amenorrhea) in females, stunted growth, loss of appetite, loss of hair, coarsening of the hair, scaly skin eruptions, irritability, double vision, skin rashes, enlargements of the liver and the spleen, headaches and dry, itchy skin. In addition, the toxicity to the nervous system from megadoses of vitamin A is well-demonstrated. It has been reported that excessive intake of vitamin A may also, over time, produce liver cancer.

Consuming large doses of vitamin D can result in nausea, loss of hair, loss of weight, vomiting, decalcification of the bones (resulting in fragile bones), drowsiness, diarrhea, headaches, hypertension, elevated cholesterol, loss of appetite and calcium deposits in the heart, kidneys and blood vessels. In addition, the damaging effects to the kidneys from an excessive intake of vitamin D have been well-demonstrated. It has been reported that excessive intake of vitamin D may also, over time, produce liver cancer.

Excess amounts of the B vitamins and vitamin C are generally excreted in the urine, prompting many authorities to suggest that supplementation with water-soluble vitamins leaves a person with nothing more than expensive urine. However, this places an inordinate amount of stress on the liver and kidneys.

Vitamin C supplementation has been controversial since Linus Pauling suggested megadoses of the vitamin be taken as a cure for the common cold. In general, medical research has not supported his claims. Vitamin C has been shown to be beneficial to performance but only in subjects who were clearly deficient in vitamin C. As noted previously, most excessive amounts of vitamin C appear in the urine. While in the body, however, megadoses of vitamin C can be harmful. Unwanted side effects from an excessive intake of vitamin C include kidney stones, diarrhea, bladder irritation, intestinal problems, destruction of red blood cells, nausea, stomach cramps, an increase in plasma cholesterol, ulceration of the gastric wall, leaching of calcium from the bones and gout. "Rebound scurvy" has also been reported after withdrawal from chronic vitamin C administration.

Excessive mineral intake. For individuals receiving the RDA of minerals, there is no evidence that mineral supplements benefit exercise performance. However, an excessive intake of minerals has the potential for adverse side effects. It should also be noted that many products contain minerals for which the National Academy of Sciences has not established RDAs. Indeed, there's no evidence that many of the minerals that are frequently listed on product labels are needed in the human body.

Herbs et al.

Many herbals and other botanical (i.e., plant-derived) products come with express or implied disease-related claims and are marketed for specific therapeutic purposes for which there may not be valid scientific support. A 1993 literature review of all the clinical trials published in the biomedical literature between 1966 and 1992 found no scientific evidence to support the

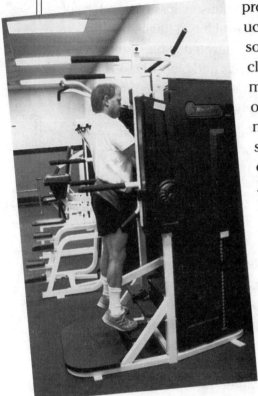

promotional claims for 42 percent of the products. Another 32 percent of the products had some scientific documentation to support their claims but were judged to be marketed in a misleading manner. In other words, 74 percent of the natural products reviewed were either marketed in a misleading fashion or had no scientific evidence to substantiate their claims. The products examined included Argentinian bull testes, boron, chromium picolinate, clenbuterol, dibencozide, plant sterols, yohimbe bark, inosine and ma huang.

The truth is that a large number of these substances have no recognized role in nutrition. Additionally, the origin and safety of many natural products remains a question. One researcher reported five cases of acute toxic hepatitis related to the use of the herb chaparral. The medical literature contains reports of severe liver toxicity linked to the widely used herb germander. Between 1985 and 1993, at least 7 cases of liver disease — with one death reported — have been associated with the oral use of products made from the leafy plant comfrey. Hypertension, rapid heart rate, nerve damage, muscle injury, psychosis, stroke and memory loss have been reported from the use of ma huang. The City of New York Department of Consumer Affairs reports that large doses of the natural stimulants found in the herb ginseng can cause hypertension, insomnia, depression and skin blemishes. Products containing yohimbine — a substance which is extracted from the inner bark of the yohimbe tree — has been linked to kidney failure, seizures and death. There are similar safety concerns with high-potency enzymes and glandular extracts from dried animal organs such as the pituitary gland, the thyroid gland and the testicles. Remember, just because a product claims to have "natural" ingredients doesn't mean that it's necessarily safe.

By the way, no known herb or any other substance can "burn" fat or facilitate its metabolism. The only real method of losing fat is exercise.

Above: The only real method of losing fat is exercise. (Photo by Matt Brzycki)

FOOD FOR THOUGHT

As long as you consume a variety of foods that provide adequate calories and nutrients, there's no need for you to take nutritional supplements. Research has concluded that nutritional supplements have little or no positive influence on performance and may even be physiologically damaging. Investing your money in high-quality foods instead of purchasing expensive nutritional supplements will result in greater success in maximizing your potential in a far safer manner. There are no shortcuts to proper nutrition.

10
Cross-Training
Activities

In order to improve your fitness, you should choose activities that require a continuous effort, are rhythmic in nature and involve large amounts of muscle mass. Additionally, the activities you select must be performed with an appropriate frequency, intensity and duration. If these three factors are similar in terms of total caloric expenditure, your physiological improvements will be the same — regardless of the activity you've chosen. Your heart doesn't know if you pedaled on a stationary cycle one day and ran on a motorized treadmill the next. The only thing that really matters is whether or not your heart received a meaningful workload. Therefore, you can use a variety of activities when cross training for fitness. In fact, variety is the trademark of cross training.

No doubt, some people will enjoy performing a variety of activities; others will savor repeating the same activity. Nevertheless, performing a variety of activities certainly reduces the potential for boredom.

Besides avoiding monotony, using different activities on a regular basis can help you to reduce your risk of experiencing or complicating an orthopedic problem. When selecting cross-training activities, it's important to distinguish between activities that are "weightbearing" from those that are "non-weightbearing." A weightbearing activity is one in which you are in direct contact with the ground so that you must support or "bear" your own bodyweight. Running and rope jumping are two classic examples of weightbearing activities. Conversely, a non-weightbearing activity is one in which your bodyweight is supported by some other means such cycling or swimming. The main advantage of non-weightbearing activities is that you can improve your level of fitness without exposing your bones, joints and connective tissue to excessive orthopedic stress. From an orthopedic perspective, it's important to include at least some non-weightbearing activities in your cross-training program on a regular basis.

If you are an athlete preparing for a specific event — such as running or swimming — the best activities to do are the ones you're going to perform in competition. If you want to become a better runner, you must primarily run; if you want to become a better swimmer, you must primarily swim. If you are a competitive runner or participate in a sport or activity that involves running — like soccer or basketball — you must use running as your primary cross-training activity. Otherwise, the best cross-training activities are the ones that are enjoyable, convenient, orthopedically safe and specific to your preparation for a sport or event.

ACTIVITIES: INDOOR vs OUTDOOR

You can perform your cross-training activities either indoors or outdoors. There are a number of general advantages and disadvantages to both indoor and outdoor activities.

Outdoor activities tend to be more fun — you can exercise in a natural environment with a variety of terrain and scenery. With indoor activities, boredom may eventually be a problem. On the other hand, most indoor equipment displays digital feedback of your performance such as your estimated speed, distance, caloric expenditure and so on. Besides making the activity more interesting, this information also enables you to quantify your workout and monitor your progress.

A disadvantage of outdoor activities is the potential for inclement weather which may force you to postpone or cancel your cross-training or to perform it under harsh or hazardous conditions. When cross training indoors, the weather isn't a factor — your indoor activities are essentially weather-proof.

As with strength training — where machines have certain advantages over free weights and vice versa — each cross-training activity has its strong and weak points. The following is a roster of the most popular cross-training activities with a candid description of both the pros and cons:

Aerobic Dancing

Since the early 1980s, aerobic-dance classes — or simply "aerobics" — have skyrocketed in popularity among fitness enthusiasts. Aerobic dancing has been crafted as an effective way of increasing fitness in large numbers of

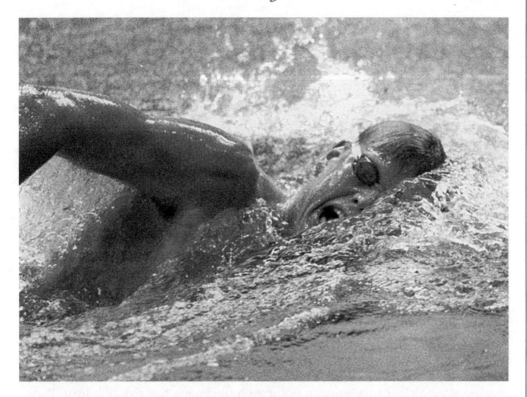

people in a pleasant, music-filled atmosphere. Aerobics is a combination of rhythmic dancing, calisthenics and flexibility movements that are blended together by the instruction of a class leader.

Aerobic dancing has a number of appealing features. Exercising to the rhythm of music makes for a more enjoyable fitness activity. Being active with a number of other participants who share a mutual goal spawns general motivation and overall enthusiasm. Monotony usually isn't a concern with aerobic dancing since classes change with the levels of difficulty, the selection of music and even the personality of instructors. A wide variety of aerobic classes are available which also reduces the possibility of boredom. For example, classes range from established, long-time favorites such as the so-called Low-Impact and Step Aerobics to newer variations that involve a variety of combative skills such as "Boxercise" and "Boxaerobics." Some aerobic classes involve the use of hand-held weights or some type of resistive bands; other classes focus entirely upon specific muscle groups such as your hips and abdominals.

Above: The main advantage of non-weightbearing activities such as swimming is that you can improve your level of fitness without exposing your bones, joints and connective tissue to excessive orthopedic stress. (Photo provided by the Princeton University office of Athletic Communications)

However, aerobic dancing has several potential problem areas. Aerobic dancing requires some degree of motor skill and coordination which may be a problem for some people — especially beginners. More than any other type of cross-training activity, the effectiveness of aerobic dancing is dependent upon an instructor and his or her skills in direction, safety and motivation. A poor class leader can mean a loss of optimal training benefits.

Perhaps the biggest concern with aerobics is that the potential for chronic and acute injuries is relatively high. A large number of injuries relating to aerobic dancing have been reported — injuries to students as well as instructors. Over the course of time, participating in classes that involve 45 - 60 minutes of high-impact activity can place an inordinate amount of stress on the knees, shins, ankles and lower back. Step aerobics places even greater orthopedic demands on the lumbar spine and lower body which — when done in excess — can quickly lead to a variety of overuse injuries. This is especially true for beginners, overweight individuals and those with a history of orthopedic problems. Low-impact aerobics — that is, keeping at least one foot on the ground at all times — reduces the amount of orthopedic stress and is a favorable alternative for the aforementioned populations. The aerobic flooring is a very important factor in reducing the risk of injury: The softer and more yielding the surface, the less orthopedic stress on your joints. Along these lines, appropriate footwear that provides cushion, support, flexibility and traction should also be worn.

Your caloric expenditure during aerobic dancing can vary considerably. Like other cross-training activities, the energy requirements for aerobic dancing are directly related to your intensity. You can increase your level of intensity during aerobics by using hand-held weights or other resistive tools, exercising at a quicker pace or performing the movements throughout a greater range of motion.

Cross-Country Skiing

An excellent low-impact activity that can be performed indoors or outdoors is cross-country skiing. An advantage of cross-country skiing is that it demands the coordinated efforts of virtually all of your major muscle groups. Because it influences such a large amount of muscle mass, your caloric expenditure can be very high — though this depends upon your level of intensity. A general disadvantage of cross-country skiing is that it can be expensive. A drawback specific to outdoor cross-country skiing is that it is a seasonal activity that requires snowy surroundings. Additionally, cross-country skiing demands some degree of proficiency and coordination.

Several devices closely simulate the action of outdoor cross-country skiing. Indoor ski machines are convenient and can provide an effective workout. One of the world's most popular indoor ski machines is the NordicTrack. This particular ski machine was invented in the mid 1970s by an engineer in a Minnesota garage. The machine was actually designed specifically for his daughter who was training for a berth on the U. S. Olympic cross-country ski team. Nearly 20 years later, this device is so popular that the name "NordicTrack" has become a generic term for any indoor ski machine.

With some indoor ski machines, the motion of the "skis" is dependent-action — the movement of one ski acts counter to the movement of the other ski. In other words, as you move one ski forward, the other ski moves backward the same distance. On other models, the skis move independently — each ski functions separately from the other. Independent-action machines provide a more realistic way to "ski."

When cross-country skiing outdoors, you can increase your intensity by skiing at a faster rate, involving more hilly terrain or wearing a weighted vest or backpack; when using an indoor ski machine, you can raise your intensity by skiing at a faster pace or increasing either the resistance level or the elevation.

Cycling

Whether it is performed indoors or outdoors, cycling is an extremely popular and productive cross-training activity. Indoor and outdoor cycling have several general advantages and disadvantages. Cycling is non-weightbearing and, therefore, can be performed in an orthopedically-safe manner. For this reason, cycling is usually included in most rehabilitation programs as one of the first activities used to "recondition" individuals and expedite their return to good health. Another general advantage of cycling is that you can target the muscles of your lower body. Perhaps the only general disadvantage of cycling is that a piece of equipment — namely a cycle — is needed.

No doubt, one of the first activities you ever learned as a child was pedaling a cycle outdoors. Outdoor cycling is a relatively inexpensive — yet healthy — form of transportation. Outdoor cycling can be done over a variety of terrains ranging from your local neighborhood to various roads and trails.

For some people, a drawback to outdoor cycling is that it requires a bit more balance and coordination than its indoor counterpart. Outdoor cycling also carries with it a relatively small but ever-present risk of injury. Regardless of the local laws, it's a good idea for you to wear protective apparel — especially headgear.

One of the most widely used pieces of exercise equipment in the United States is the indoor or "stationary" cycle. There are several advantages of using a stationary cycle. First of all, there's no balance or coordination needed for stationary cycling. Further, stationary cycling requires no special skill because the rotary motion is the same no matter what type of cycle you pedal. In addition, stationary cycles are relatively simple to operate. Finally, you can use a few different cross-training methods when pedaling a stationary cycle — from continuous aerobic efforts to intermittent anaerobic work.

Some stationary cycles provide you with the option of doing upper-body ergometry or, more simply, exercise for your upper torso. Equipment that permits upper-body exercise is advantageous for several reasons. Suppose you sustained an injury to your lower body that prohibited you from doing any cross-training activity that involved your hips and legs. Having access to equipment that provides upper-body exercise allows you to continue your cross training in spite of your unfortunate injury. Additionally, performing synchronous activity for your upper and lower bodies allows you to use calories at a greater rate. Finally, equipment that lets you exercise your upper torso and lower body offers increased variety: You can exercise with just your legs, just your arms or both your arms and your legs. (It's important to note that, generally speaking, your upper-body muscles have less strength, endurance and mass than your lower-body muscles. When exercising smaller muscles, less fibers are available to "share" the workload. Because of this, your heart-rate and blood-pressure responses are higher for activities involving your upper body than activities involving your lower body at the same level of intensity. In other words, the physiological demands are greater at the same level of intensity when using smaller muscles.)

A stationary cycle usually resembles a traditional outdoor cycle in that the user is in an upright position. A recent innovation that is quickly gaining favor among fitness enthusiasts is the "recumbent cycle." When using this particular cycle, you are positioned in a wide, car-like bucket-seat with your feet in front of you (rather than underneath you). Compared to a traditional upright position, a recumbent position enhances comfort dramatically and also reduces the stress on the lumbar spine. Recumbent cycles are especially comfortable for populations with special needs including older adults, overweight individuals, pregnant females and those with chronic low-back pain.

Whether you are cycling indoors or outdoors, the seat should be adjusted so that your legs are almost completely extended at the bottom of the pedaling stroke. In addition, the use of toe clips will improve your pedaling efficiency.

With outdoor cycling, you can increase your intensity by pedaling at a faster pace, using a more difficult gear or involving more hilly terrain; when cycling indoors, you can raise your intensity by cycling at a faster pace or increasing the level of tension.

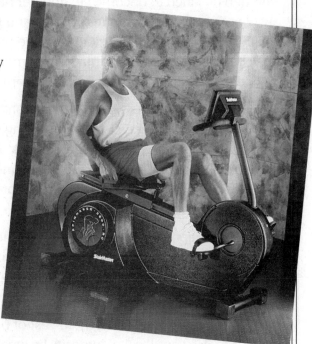

Hiking/Backpacking

Hiking and backpacking have the same favorable attributes as most other outdoor activities. Your activities can range from a leisurely stroll over a hilly path to an adventurous trek over a mountainous trail. Though technically considered to be weightbearing activities, hiking and backpacking involve much lower impact forces and, therefore, expose your body to less orthopedic stress than other weightbearing activities that have higher impact forces such as running.

Your caloric expenditure during hiking and backpacking is a function of the terrain, packloads and altitude. You can increase your intensity while hiking and backpacking by wearing a heavier backpack or weighted vest, walking at a faster pace or using steeper grades.

Ice/In-Line (or Roller) Skating

Another cross-training activity that is extremely popular and enjoyable is skating. Whether it is done on ice or pavement, skating is an excellent low-impact activity for your hips and legs — particularly your inner and outer thigh. Because skating involves horizontal leg action (rather than vertical), the impact forces are virtually eliminated. One of the disadvantages of skating, however, is that it demands a certain amount of balance, coordination and skill.

In the early 1980s, Minnesotan Scott Olson built the first pair of "Rollerblades." When first introduced to the fitness scene, in-line skating

Above: Recumbent cycles are especially comfortable for populations with special needs including older adults, overweight individuals, pregnant females and those with chronic low-back pain. (Photo provided by StairMaster Sports/ Medical Products, Inc.)

seemed destined to become yet another passing fad. However, the popularity of in-line skating continues to grow and seems here to stay. In fact, in-line skating has replaced roller skating as the preferred method of skating on a paved surface. It's been estimated that more than 30 million people utilize in-line skates during activities ranging from in-line skating to roller hockey.

In a 1996 study, university researchers concluded that "in-line skating is an appropriate form of exercise for improving cardiovascular fitness." However, in-line skating carries some degree of risk. In 1994, the cost of emergency room treatment due to in-line skating injuries was estimated at $346 million. Therefore, it's very critical that you wear protective gear including a helmet, elbow pads and wrist guards.

With the exception of performing within the confines of a rink, skating is primarily an outdoor activity. Nautilus International has developed a machine that takes up very little space and approximates the action of skating.

You can increase your intensity during ice and in-line skating by using a faster pace or wearing a weighted vest or backpack; with in-line skating, you can also raise your level of intensity by involving steeper grades.

Rope Jumping

There are a few advantages to jumping rope. For one thing, rope jumping is inexpensive. In addition, it is portable and can be performed just about anywhere.

Rope jumping has a few drawbacks. In order to produce adequate benefits, you must have a fair amount of proficiency at jumping rope. Although rope jumping exercises your upper and lower bodies simultaneously, it sometimes involves a relatively small amount of muscle mass: your calves and forearms.

The biggest disadvantage of rope jumping is that it is a high-impact activity. Compared to low-impact and non-weightbearing activities, jumping rope has a higher risk of excessive orthopedic stress — particularly to the ankles, knees and lower back — and a greater potential for overuse injuries. Some populations are at a greater risk than others. For instance, larger-than-average people (larger due to either fat tissue or muscle tissue) experience more pounding of their joints than smaller individuals. In addition, a woman who jumps rope during her pregnancy may endanger her fetus. Jumping rope shouldn't be done in the early stages of your cross-training program, either.

The best ropes have handles containing ball bearings which make the effort easier and smoother. Like all other high-impact activities, good footwear that has adequate cushion and support provide important shock-absorbing qualities.

When jumping rope, you can increase your intensity by jumping at a faster pace; if you alternate your feet, you can raise your level of intensity by moving your legs through a greater range of motion.

Rowing

The coordinated efforts of nearly all of your major muscle groups — that is, your hips, legs, lower back and the pulling muscles of your upper torso — are involved in rowing. Exercising continuously with this large amount of muscle mass creates a sizable expenditure of calories. A disadvantage of outdoor rowing is the need for an accessible body of water that is suitable for rowing.

Rowing is an excellent outdoor activity but it is equally effective when done indoors. In 1987, the first indoor rowing "regatta" was organized by a group of former rowers who competed as members of the United States National Team. In honor of their previous athletic experiences, the event was labeled "CRASH-B" which stood for "Charles River All Star Has-Beens." Since then, indoor rowing competitions have grown throughout the world and involve thousands of participants. Unfortunately, few companies manufacture an indoor rower that gives a true simulation or feeling of actually pulling an oar through water. Among competitive and recreational rowers, the most popu-

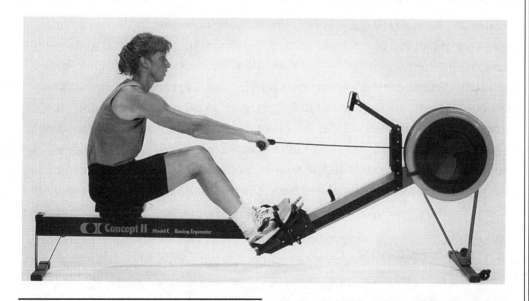

Above: The coordinated efforts of nearly all of your major muscle groups — that is, your hips, legs, lower back and the pulling muscles of your upper torso — are involved in rowing. (Photo provided by Concept II, Inc.)

lar indoor rower is the "Concept II" rowing ergometer or "erg." (An ergo-meter is a device that measures work.)

To obtain maximum benefits and reduce your risk of injury, it's important to row with proper technique. Whether you are outdoors or indoors, you should begin the "drive" phase of the rowing movement by using your powerful hip, leg and low-back muscles and finish the stroke by pulling the handle to your mid-section with your arms. At the end of the stroke, your legs should be straight and you should be leaning slightly backward. The "recovery" phase is done in the reverse order, starting by extending your arms and then bringing your torso forward using your hips and legs. Those with low-back problems should probably pursue other cross-training activities.

With outdoor rowing, you can increase your intensity by rowing at a faster pace or rowing against a current; when rowing indoors, you can elevate your intensity by rowing at a faster rate or increasing the level of resistance.

Stair Climbing/Stepping

In 1984, the era of stair-climbing machines began at a Chicago trade show in a vendor booth that measured a meager 8 x 10 feet. Despite this rather anonymous and humble beginning, the popularity of these machines has grown steadily since the latter part of the 1980s. In fact, the use of stair-climbing machines may have more widespread appeal than any other cross-training tool that is used in the commercial and residential settings.

There are basically two kinds of stair climbers: One type has a revolving staircase while the other features two steps on which you stand and exer-cise. There are two categories of "two-step" models: dependent and inde-pendent. With a dependent-action stair climber, the movement of one step is counter to the movement of the other step. In other words, as one step goes down a certain distance, the other automatically comes up the same distance. With an independent-action stair climber, each step operates separately from the other. Some stair-climbing machines also provide activ-ity for the muscles of your upper body. (The advantages of equipment that offers the option of upper-body activity are noted under "Cycling.")

 When used correctly, stair-climbing machines can be extremely productive and physically demanding. Stair climbers are fairly easy to operate and allow for different methods of cross training — ranging from continuous aerobic activity to intermittent anaerobic efforts. In general, stair-climbing machines provide low-impact activity since your feet never leave the ground.

On the downside, many stair-climbing machines are of poor quality and may not be very durable. If you're buying a stair climber for personal use, the cost can be a prohibiting factor. Another disadvantage of stair-climbing machines is the absolute need to utilize proper technique. The device should be used without supporting a portion of your bodyweight on the handrail or the front of the machine. When you "off-load" in this manner, the activity is less effective and your performance estimates (i.e., your caloric expenditure, floors climbed and so on) can be inflated — sometimes significantly. In addition, the contorted body position from off-loading increases your risk of injury due to improper

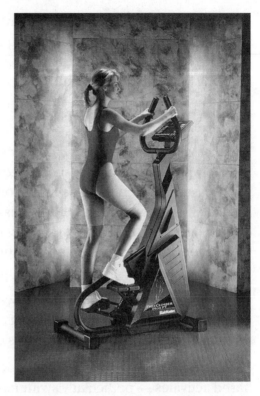

and unnatural body mechanics. More importantly, however, is the fact that some stair-climbing machines are poorly designed and may predispose the knee to hyperextension at the bottom portion of the movement. In particular, your knees are exposed to high levels of orthopedic stress when using dependent-action stair climbers. The safest stair climbers to use are the ones in which the surface of the steps remain parallel to the floor throughout their travel. The most popular stair climber in the world is the StairMaster — a name that has become a general term for any type of stair-climbing machine.

An effective alternative that is closely related to mechanical stair-climbing machines is bench stepping. Bench stepping can be done in your home with little or no equipment — you can simply climb up and down a staircase or several aerobic steps stacked on the floor. Similarly, the outdoor equivalent of indoor bench stepping is walking up and down stadium bleachers. A disadvantage of bench stepping is that it is a high-impact activity because your feet leave the ground. Another disadvantage of bench stepping is the potential for boredom.

Above: The use of stair-climbing machines may have more widespread appeal than any other cross-training tool that is used in the commercial and residential settings. (Photo provided by StairMaster Sports/Medical Products, Inc.)

You can raise your intensity during any stair-climbing activity by wearing a weighted backpack or vest, increasing the height of your steps or stepping more rapidly. It is important to note that wearing extra weight during stair-climbing activities should be done infrequently and in moderation since this increases the orthopedic stress.

Swimming/Aquatic Exercising

The idea of using water-based movements as cross-training activities was probably popularized by the sportsmedical community. It was found that, in many cases, individuals with chronic orthopedic problems or recent musculoskeletal injuries could usually exercise in water with little or no associated orthopedic discomfort. The swimming pool has since emerged as a new frontier for conditioning healthy, uninjured individuals.

Several aquatic activities can be done in the shallow end of the pool such as walking/jogging/running through the water, calisthenics and "aqua-aerobic" classes. However, the most popular of all aquatic activities is swimming. A number of different swimming strokes can be used in the pool.

There are many advantages to aquatic activities. For example, many water-based activities — particularly swimming — involve the simultaneous usage of your upper- and lower-body musculature. This large amount of muscle mass requires high levels of caloric expenditure. More importantly, swimming and other activities done in an aquatic environment are non-weightbearing which virtually eliminates the compressive forces on your bones, joints and connective tissue. Since your bodyweight is supported by the water, aquatic activities have a lower potential for musculoskeletal injuries than traditional weightbearing activities.

A drawback of aquatic activities is that some individuals may not be comfortable around water. In addition, you must have access to a swimming pool.

There are several downsides that are specific to swimming. For one, swimming requires a relatively higher level of motor skill than other activities like stationary cycling or rowing. A highly specialized skill like swimming may take a considerable amount of practice to master. As such, a lack of adequate swimming skills can interfere with your potential cross-training benefits. If you have a low level of fitness or have poor swimming skills, your exercising heart rate may exceed your recommended training zone in a struggle just to keep yourself afloat. If you aren't accustomed to swimming or skilled at it, you'll also tire very quickly. Therefore, swimming isn't a good aerobic option for anyone with poor swimming fundamentals. However, swimming represents an excellent choice if your skills are adequate. Flotation devices — such as an aqua-vest or a simple kick-board — can help overcome any shortcomings of swimming skills.

Your caloric expenditure during swimming is influenced by a number of factors including your speed of movement, the stroke you use and even the water temperature. Your caloric expenditure is also highly related to your level of skill. A skilled swimmer requires less energy to move through the water. In fact, an unskilled swimmer may use twice as many calories to maintain the same velocity as a skilled swimmer.

The amount of work you do in relation to your caloric expenditure is referred to as your biomechanical efficiency. Women tend to be more efficient swimmers than men partly because of their greater body-fat stores as well as a more even distribution of body fat which improves buoyancy. (Flotation devices can also enhance buoyancy.)

Your heart-rate response while swimming at a specific oxygen intake is about 14 beats per minute lower than running at the same level of oxygen intake. The diminished cardiac work is due to exercising in the prone position and the effect of being immersed in a relatively cool environment. Therefore, your heart-rate training zone should be slightly lower during swimming compared to other cross-training activities. You can increase your intensity during stationary aquatic activities by using devices to resist your movements such as hand-bar exercisers, hand paddles, webbed gloves and kick-boards; your intensity can be raised while swimming by moving at a faster pace or by pulling resistive devices through the water such as buoy blocks.

Walking/Jogging/Running

Few cross-training activities enjoy such world-wide popularity as walking/jogging/running outdoors. These activities are so appealing because they are simple and natural: No special equipment, elaborate machine, unique clothing or new skill is necessary for a productive workout.

The main characteristic that distinguishes walking from jogging and running is biomechanical: When walking, at least one foot is in contact with the ground at all times; when jogging and running, the body is propelled completely off the ground. Essentially, the difference between jogging and running is the speed. Jogging is basically slower running. In order to simplify matters, most of the following discussion uses "running" as an umbrella term for "jogging and running."

The preferred cross-training activity of many individuals is walking. It is perhaps the most basic, natural, practical and enjoyable activity of all. Walking is also convenient: Given sufficient space, walking can be done almost anywhere — indoors or outdoors. It is often chosen because of its relatively low injury-rate, simplicity and adaptability to busy schedules. Walking can be especially beneficial for sedentary or overweight individuals or those with a low level of fitness. To avoid injury, appropriate footwear is very important. Specialized walking shoes are available but you can simply use footwear that is comfortable and durable and offers plenty of support.

Jogging is a natural progression from walking; running is a natural progression from jogging. Most of the advantages of walking also apply to jogging and running. Like all weightbearing activities, however, one of the drawbacks of jogging and running is the potential for overuse injury and other orthopedic problems. This is especially relevant for beginners and larger individuals — larger due to either fat tissue or muscle tissue — who subject their bones, joints and connective tissue to a large amount of stress when running. There's no question that running is a high-impact activity: It has been estimated that your lower extremities absorb 2 - 3 times your bodyweight when running. So, a person weighing 170 pounds must dissipate roughly 340 - 510 pounds of downward force that occurs with each footfall — and there may be 1,000 footfalls per mile. There is a greater potential for injury when jogging or running on hard surfaces. However, jogging or running on a yielding surface such as grass or a motorized treadmill reduces the impact forces. You can reduce your risk of orthopedic problems even further by regularly alternating non-weightbearing activities with your jogging and running.

When jogging or running, it is important to use footwear that is comfortable and durable. Proper footwear can act as a shock-absorber and soften the associated impact forces. Therefore, appropriate shoes should also provide adequate cushion, good heel support and sufficient mid-sole flexibility.

Generally speaking, your caloric expenditure while walking at slower speeds is relatively low compared to jogging or running. However, the caloric cost of walking at 5 miles per hour or faster approaches that of jogging and running.

One of the most preferred pieces of indoor cross-training equipment is the treadmill. There are basically two types of treadmills: motorized and self-propelled. Treadmills that are motor-driven tend to be of far better quality than their self-propelled counterparts. Walking, jogging or running on a treadmill provides exactly the same fitness benefits as those of their outdoor counterparts. Furthermore, many of the advantages of activities done on a treadmill are the same as those of similar outdoor activities. In addition, treadmills offer fingertip control of your speed and digital estimates of your performance. Many treadmills also

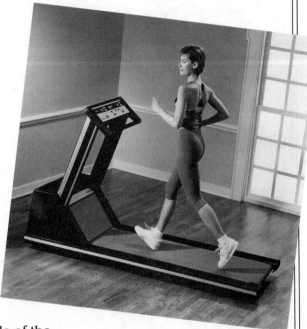

allow you to easily adjust the angle of the tread to either inclined or declined grades which simulates moving uphill or downhill. Another advantage of a treadmill is that your running can be done indoors in a controlled environment that is constant and comfortable. When walking/jogging/running on a treadmill indoors, there's no need to worry about uneven surfaces, traffic, pollution or exhaust fumes from vehicles. Finally, many newer models offer some type of shock-absorbing component beneath the tread which lessens the impact forces.

On the downside, a high-quality motorized treadmill is probably the most expensive of all cross-training tools. Another disadvantage is the risk of losing your balance or falling off the back of the tread while exercising.

The intensity of walking, jogging and running can be increased by moving at a faster pace or involving steeper inclines; when walking, you can also raise your level of intensity by wearing a backpack or weighted vest or carrying light hand-held weights. (Jogging or running with extra weight increases the orthopedic stress and isn't advisable.)

Above: One of the most preferred pieces of indoor cross-training equipment is the motorized treadmill. (Photo provided by Quinton Fitness Equipment)

11

Six-Month Sample Cross-Training Program

A cross-training program can be structured an infinite number of ways. It's literally impossible to specify one cross-training program that is ideally suited for everyone. The structure of your cross-training program depends upon several personal factors including your level of fitness, individual preferences, orthopedic concerns, convenience and availability of equipment. Nevertheless, there are certain common elements that everyone must consider.

VARIETY

In order to combat the boredom and drudgery associated with performing the same activity day after day for long periods of time, it's important for you to vary your cross-training program on a regular basis. There are many variables that you can manipulate such as the duration of your workout, the frequency of your training and your level of intensity. One of the simplest ways of varying your program is to alternate your activities from one day to the next. As an example, your three weekly workouts can include one day of cycling, one day of running and one day of swimming. You can also combine several different activities within a single workout. For instance, you might do 10 minutes of cycling, 10 minutes of rowing and 10 minutes of stair climbing for a total of 30 minutes of cross-training exercise. Instead of focusing on the duration of your activity, you can also use caloric expenditure as a target. For example, your goal might be to expend a total of 300 calories: 100 calories while cycling, 100 calories while rowing and 100 calories while stair climbing.

Rather than alternating your cross-training activities daily, you may prefer to do it weekly or monthly. Or, you can simply vary your cross-training activities at random. (Keep in mind that you should take time off regularly.)

To reduce your risk of orthopedic stress, you might alternate weightbearing and non-weightbearing activities. If you have existing orthopedic concerns, you should avoid weightbearing activities — especially those that involve high-impact forces.

SCHEDULING TRAINING SESSIONS

You must determine the most practical way of scheduling your workouts for strength training and conditioning (i.e., aerobic and/or anaerobic). This may be done two different ways: You can perform both activities on the same day or on alternate days. The advantage of doing both activities on the same day is that it permits a more complete recovery. If you do your strength training on one day and your conditioning the next, your muscles will be constantly stressed and may not have adequate time to recover properly. After a while, it may also be very difficult for you to perform intensive training sessions several days in a row without a break with a high-degree of enthusiasm. Therefore, the recommended way for you to schedule your strength training and conditioning sessions is to do both activities on the same day. For example, a 60-minute workout might include 30 minutes of conditioning and 30 minutes of strength training or 40 minutes of conditioning and 20 minutes of strength training. If you don't have enough time to perform both activities on the same day, you can do the activities on alternating days.

SEQUENCE OF ACTIVITIES

It's important for all individuals to improve their levels of strength and fitness. Competitive athletes must be also concerned with improving their sport-specific skills. If you must perform your skill work, conditioning and strength training on the same day, you'll obtain better results if you do your skill work first. Of all three activities, the one that is most critical to an athlete is skill development. If you're exhausted after your conditioning and strength training, you'll be drained both physically and mentally. Therefore, you won't practice very hard or work on your technique very well. In fact, you're sure to be inattentive and your performance will probably be quite careless, labored and awkward. Furthermore, you're more prone to injury when you practice in a pre-fatigued state. Because of this, it's best that you don't practice your athletic skills after performing intense strength training and/or conditioning activities.

After completing their skill training, athletes can either perform their strength training followed by their conditioning or their conditioning followed by their strength training. The activity that should be done first depends upon the nature of their sport. If their sport has a greater strength component — such as shot putting and high jumping — then those athletes should perform their strength-training workout before their conditioning workout. On the other hand, if their sport has a greater endurance component — such as basketball and soccer — then their conditioning workout should precede their strength-training workout.

But what if you're not a competitive athlete? If increasing muscular strength is your primary goal then you should perform your strength training before your conditioning; if improving your aerobic fitness is your main objective then you should do your conditioning before your strength training.

Research indicates that better overall results are obtained when conditioning activities are performed before strength-training activities. In a 1986 study, subjects performed a strength-training workout, rested for 5 minutes and then cycled for 20 minutes of aerobic activity. During a subsequent session, the same subjects cycled for 20 minutes of aerobic activity, rested for 5 minutes and then performed a strength training workout. Performing the strength-training workout before the conditioning workout resulted in a 1-percent improvement in strength performance compared to performing the strength-training workout after the conditioning workout; performing the conditioning workout before the strength-training workout resulted in an 8-percent improvement in conditioning performance compared to performing the conditioning workout after the strength-training workout. The study also suggested that strength training has a greater impact on aerobic conditioning performance than aerobic conditioning has on strength performance.

A SAMPLE PROGRAM

The following example isn't intended to be an optimal cross-training program. Rather, it should be used only as a guideline to help you craft your own personal cross-training program. You should adjust the design of your program to meet your own personal interests and functional abilities.

This six-month sample program specifies three cross-training sessions per week on non-consecutive days. Though not mentioned in the monthly plans, strength-training activities should also be scheduled 2 - 3 times per week. Whether you perform your strength training on the same days as your aerobic cross training or on alternate days is your choice. Warming up and stretching aren't indicated in the monthly plans either but should be done prior to activities that involve rapid muscle contractions — such as sprinting — in order to reduce your risk of injury.

MONTH 1

During the initial stages of your cross-training program, you should concentrate on several basic activities. In the first two weeks of this example, the cross-training activities are simply stair climbing and running. A new activity is introduced during the third week: outdoor cycling. Performing an unfamiliar activity will probably result in some muscle soreness for a day or two after exercise. However, any soreness will disappear once your body has grown accustomed to the activity. In the early part of your cross training, it's especially important that you don't perform your activities for an excessive amount of time as a precaution against overuse injury. Along these lines, note that in this example a high-impact, weightbearing activity — that is, running — has only been scheduled once per week to reduce the risk of orthopedic problems.

Week One	
Mon	15:00 stair climbing
Wed	15:00 running
Fri	15:00 stair climbing

Week Two	
Mon	16:00 stair climbing
Wed	16:00 running
Fri	16:00 stair climbing

Week Three	
Mon	15:00 outdoor cycling
Wed	17:00 running
Fri	17:00 stair climbing

Week Four	
Mon	16:00 outdoor cycling
Wed	17:00 running
Fri	18:00 stair climbing

MONTH 2

The first week of this month adds another activity: indoor rowing. This cross-training activity involves exercise for the upper-torso musculature. Keep in mind that when you exercise different muscles than usual, it will probably cause some degree of muscle soreness. Furthermore, performing additional exercise for the upper-body muscles — as in the case of indoor rowing — may initially have an adverse impact upon the performance of those specific muscles in strength-training activities. As a training variation, cycling is moved indoors during this second month. The third week of the month introduces indoor cross-country skiing as a new activity.

Week One	
Mon	15:00 indoor rowing
Wed	18:00 running
Fri	17:00 indoor cycling

Week Two	
Mon	16:00 indoor rowing
Wed	18:00 running
Fri	18:00 indoor cycling

Week Three	
Mon	15:00 indoor skiing
Wed	19:00 running
Fri	17:00 indoor rowing

Week Four	
Mon	16:00 indoor skiing
Wed	19:00 running
Fri	18:00 indoor rowing

MONTH 3

No new cross-training activities are introduced during the third month of this fictional program. Rather, the weekly sequences and combinations of familiar activities are merely rearranged to provide variety.

Week One	
Mon	17:00 stair climbing
Wed	20:00 running
Fri	17:00 indoor skiing

Week Two	
Mon	18:00 stair climbing
Wed	20:00 running
Fri	18:00 indoor skiing

Week Three	
Mon	17:00 indoor rowing
Wed	21:00 running
Fri	19:00 stair climbing

Week Four	
Mon	18:00 indoor rowing
Wed	21:00 running
Fri	20:00 stair climbing

MONTH 4

The fourth month begins with a week in which no cross-training activities are scheduled. Taking time off periodically from your cross-training activities can help you avoid overtraining. In the second week, a simple variation in training is made by moving the cycling back to an outdoor setting. Also in the second week, swimming replaces running as the mid-week activity. Essentially, this exchanges a high-impact, weightbearing activity for one that is low-impact and non-weightbearing to allow for a prolonged period of reduced orthopedic stress. As noted previously, any muscle soreness that may result from performing a new activity will dissipate once your muscles become familiar with the unaccustomed actions.

Week One	
Mon	no cross-training activity
Wed	no cross-training activity
Fri	no cross-training activity

Week Two	
Mon	19:00 outdoor cycling
Wed	15:00 swimming
Fri	19:00 indoor skiing

Week Three	
Mon	20:00 indoor skiing
Wed	16:00 swimming
Fri	18:00 indoor rowing

Week Four	
Mon	20:00 indoor skiing
Wed	17:00 swimming
Fri	19:00 indoor rowing

MONTH 5

During the first week of this month, a basic form of Circuit Aerobic Training (CAT) is introduced. The CAT is scheduled once per week and, for variety, uses four different combinations of familiar cross-training activities. Note that the combinations pair two activities — one of which provides upper-body exercise. Running is also reintroduced as the mid-week activity.

Week One	
Mon	10:00 stair climbing + 10:00 indoor rowing
Wed	18:00 running
Fri	18:00 swimming

Week Two	
Mon	10:00 indoor cycling + 10:00 indoor skiing
Wed	18:00 running
Fri	19:00 swimming

Week Three	
Mon	11:00 stair climbing + 11:00 indoor skiing
Wed	19:00 running
Fri	19:00 swimming

Week Four	
Mon	11:00 indoor cycling + 11:00 indoor rowing
Wed	19:00 running
Fri	20:00 swimming

MONTH 6

Several new variations are made to the CAT that was introduced during the previous month. In the first and third weeks of this month, the CAT involves different combinations of three activities. In the fourth week, the CAT includes two activities but one is repeated a second time (i.e., cycling). Note that in all cases, the CAT alternates activities that only involve the lower body with activities that involve exercise for both the upper and lower body. A new cross-training activity is added in the third week: recumbent cycling.

Week One	
Mon	7:00 stair climbing + 7:00 indoor rowing + 7:00 indoor cycling
Wed	20:00 running
Fri	20:00 swimming

Week Two	
Mon	11:30 indoor rowing + 11:30 stair climbing
Wed	20:00 running
Fri	21:00 swimming

Week Three	
Mon	7:30 indoor skiing + 7:30 indoor cycling + 7:30 indoor rowing
Wed	21:00 running
Fri	20:00 recumbent cycling

Week Four	
Mon	8:00 indoor cycling + 8:00 indoor rowing + 8:00 indoor cycling
Wed	21:00 running
Fri	21:00 recumbent cycling

12
Cross-Training Q & A

There are some final random topics and issues that should be addressed. This chapter examines 20 of the most frequently asked questions concerning the performance of your cross-training activities.

1. How should I breathe when I lift weights?

It's important for you to breath properly when you perform a strenuous activity such as strength training — especially during maximal efforts. Holding your breath during exertion creates an elevated pressure in your abdominal and thoracic cavities which is referred to as the "Valsalva maneuver." The elevated pressure interferes with the return of blood to your heart. This may deprive your brain of blood and can cause you to lose consciousness.

To emphasize correct breathing, exhale when you raise the resistance and inhale when you lower the resistance. Or, simply remember EOE — Exhale On Effort. As it turns out, inhaling and exhaling naturally usually results in correct breathing.

2. What's the best exercise for getting rid of the "spare tire" around my mid-section?

In exercise-physiology parlance, the belief that exercise causes a localized loss of body fat is known as "spot reduction." A litmus test for evaluating the prospect of spot reduction is to examine whether a significantly greater change occurs in an active or exercised body part compared to a relatively inactive or unexercised body part. A study published in 1971 compared the circumference and the thickness of subcutaneous fat at specific sites on both arms of a group of tennis players. The use of these particular athletes

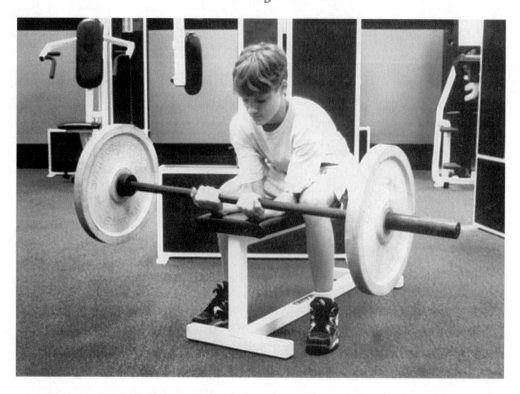

as subjects in this study is important since tennis players have subjected one side of their bodies to a significantly greater amount of exercise and activity than the other side of their bodies over a number of years. As would be expected, the study noted that both the upper and the lower arms on the more active side of the body were significantly more hypertrophied than the upper and the lower arms on the less active side of the body. However, there was no significant difference in the thickness of subcutaneous fat over the muscles of the arm receiving more exercise as compared to the arm receiving less exercise. This study provides direct evidence against the notion of spot reduction.

The abdominal area probably receives more attention than any other body part. Many people perform countless repetitions of sit-ups, knee-ups and other abdominal exercises every day with the belief that this will give them a highly prized set of "washboard abs." Although such Olympian efforts certainly work your underlying abdominal muscles, it has little effect on your overlying fatty tissue. The reason you can't lose fat in one area alone is because during exercise, energy stores from throughout your body are being

Above: To emphasize correct breathing, exhale when you raise the resistance and inhale when you lower the resistance. (Photo by Matt Brzycki)

used as a source of fuel — not just from one specific area. So, you can do endless abdominal exercises, but that won't automatically trim your mid-section. A study published in 1984 evaluated the effects of a 27-day sit-up exercise program on the fat-cell diameter and body composition of 13 subjects. Over this 4-week period, each subject performed a total of 5,004 sit-ups (with the knees flexed at 90 degrees and no foot support). Fat biopsies from the abdomen, subscapular and gluteal sites revealed that the sit-up exercise regimen reduced the fat-cell diameter at all three sites to a similar degree. In other words, exercising the underlying abdominal musculature did not preferentially effect the subcutaneous fatty layer in the abdominal region more than the buttocks or the subscapular areas. Quite simply, spot reduction is physiologically impossible.

Your abdominals should be treated like any other muscle group. Once an activity for your abdominals exceeds about 70 seconds in duration, it becomes a test of endurance rather than strength. Your abdominals can be fatigued effectively in a time-efficient manner by exercising them to the point of concentric muscular fatigue within 8 - 12 repetitions (or about 40 - 70 seconds).

3. How does my muscle-fiber type distribution influence my response to a strength-training program?

Your predominant muscle-fiber type plays a major role in determining your potential for attaining muscular size and strength. The two major types of muscle fibers are fast twitch (FT) and slow twitch (ST). Both FT and ST muscle fibers have the potential to "hypertrophy" or increase in size. (A decrease in muscle size is known as "atrophy.") However, FT fibers display a much greater capacity for hypertrophy than ST fibers. This means that people who have inherited a high percentage of FT fibers have a greater potential to increase the size of their muscles. Because FT fibers can produce greater force than ST fibers, these individuals also display a higher potential for strength gains. It's interesting to note that FT fibers not only hypertrophy faster and to a greater degree than ST fibers but also atrophy faster and to a greater extent.

No conclusive evidence exists to suggest that strength training can change ST fibers to FT fibers or vice versa. Though one type of muscle fiber may take on certain metabolic characteristics of the other type of fiber, actual conversion appears to be impossible. In other words, you cannot convert one fiber type into another any more than you can make a racehorse out of a mule. So, if you train a mule like a racehorse, you might get a faster mule but you'll never get a racehorse. For all practical purposes, your muscle-fiber composition is determined entirely by hereditary factors. Finally, there's no definitive proof that strength training increases the number of muscle fibers in humans. An increase in the number of muscle fibers — known as "hyper-plasia" — has been demonstrated in some animals but not in humans.

4. How can I avoid getting shin splints?

"Shin splints" is a general term used to describe a variety of painful condi-tions on the front part of the lower leg. The pain — often characterized as a dull ache — is usually located on the lower two-thirds of the tibia (the shin bone) and is felt during dorsi flexion and plantar flexion.

Shin splints are considered to be an overuse injury and, in general, have two main causes. In some cases, there's a strength imbalance between the muscles of the lower leg. Specifically, the "dorsi flexors" on the anterior part of the lower leg are weaker than the calf muscles on the posterior part of the leg. This situation can be remedied by performing exercises for the dorsi flexors and reducing exercises for the calves. Shin splints can also result from high-impact forces that exceed the structural integrity of the lower leg. There are a number of ways to reduce this orthopedic stress. First of all, proper shoes should be worn that provide adequate support and shock-absorbing qualities. It's also important to reduce the amount of weightbearing activities and incorporate more non-weightbearing ones. If possible, weightbearing activities should be performed on softer, more yielding surfaces.

If you have shin splints, the pain and swelling can be alleviated by applying ice to your lower-leg area. The ice treatment should last about 20 minutes and should be done as soon as possible after you've completed your cross-training activities.

5. When I stop lifting weights my muscles will turn to fat, right?

Wrong. It's a common misconception that muscle can be turned into fat. In truth, muscle cannot be changed into fat — or vice versa — any more than lead can be changed into gold. Your muscle tissue consists of special con-tractile proteins that allow movement to occur. The composition of muscle tissue is about 70-percent water, 22-percent protein and 7-percent fat. Con-versely, your fatty tissue is composed of spherical cells that are specifically designed to store fat. Fatty tissue is about 22-percent water, 6-percent protein

---

Left: A strength imbalance between the muscles of the lower leg can be remedied by performing exercises for the dorsi flexors (pictured) and reducing exercises for the calves. (Photo by Matt Brzycki)

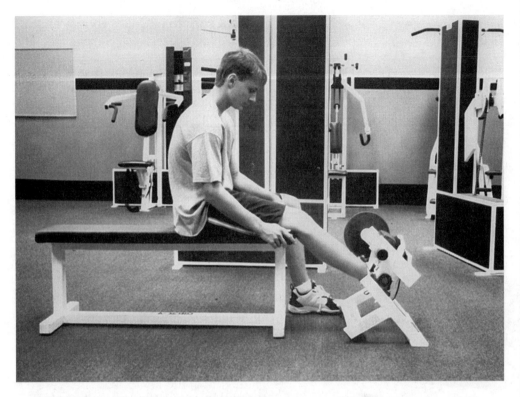

and 72-percent fat. Since muscle and fat are two different and distinct types of biological tissue, your muscles can't convert to fat if you stop lifting weights. Similarly, lifting weights — or doing any other rigorous activity — won't change your fat into muscle. The fact is that muscles atrophy (or become smaller) from prolonged disuse and muscles hypertrophy (or get larger) as a result of physical exercise.

6. How often should I max out to check my progress in the weight room?

There's no need for you to "max out" or determine how much weight you can lift for a one-repetition maximum (1-RM). Attempting to see how much weight you can lift for a 1-RM is potentially dangerous. Performing a 1-RM with heavy weights places an inordinate and unreasonable amount of stress on the muscles, bones and connective tissue. An injury occurs when this stress exceeds the structural integrity of those components. A 1-RM attempt also tends to cause an abnormally high increase in blood pressure — which may be dangerous for individuals with hypertension. Finally, a 1-RM is a highly specialized skill that requires a great deal of technique and practice.

Performing a 1-RM isn't really necessary to monitor your progress. If you are recording your workout data — and you should — you can simply check

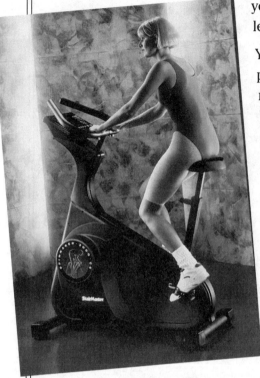

your workout card to evaluate your strength levels.

You can estimate your 1-RM in a safe and practical — yet reasonably accurate — manner without having to "max out." There's a direct relationship between the percentage of maximal load (strength) and repetitions-to-fatigue (anaerobic endurance): As the percentage of maximal weight increases, the number of repetitions decreases in an almost linear fashion. Unless you have an injury or other musculoskeletal disorder, the kinship between your muscular strength and your anaerobic endurance remains constant. Since there is a distinct relationship between these two variables, your anaerobic endurance can be determined by measuring your strength . . . and your strength can also be determined by measuring your anaerobic endurance.

This relationship is not exactly linear but it's close enough to determine a reasonably accurate linear approximation for describing the relationship between the two variables. In fact, the following mathematical equation can be used to predict a 1-RM based upon repetitions-to-fatigue:

$$\textbf{Predicted 1-RM} = \frac{\text{Weight Lifted}}{1.0278 - .0278X}$$

where x = the number of repetitions performed

Example: Suppose that you did 8 repetitions-to-fatigue with 150 pounds. First, multiplying .0278 by the number of repetitions [8] equals .2224. Subtracting .2224 from 1.0278 leaves .8054. Dividing the weight you lifted [150 pounds] by .8054 yields a predicted 1-RM of about 186 pounds.

In other words, you can do 8 repetitions with about 80.54 percent (or .8054) of your predicted 1-RM. Regardless of whether your strength increases or

Above: The most obvious indicator of overtraining is a lack of progress in your muscular strength and/or aerobic fitness. (Photo provided by StairMaster Sports/Medical Products, Inc.)

decreases, you'll always be able to perform exactly 8 repetitions with roughly 80.54 percent of your maximum. Therefore, if you increase your 8-RM (your anaerobic endurance) by 20 percent [from 150 to 180 pounds] then you'll also increase your 1-RM (your muscular strength) by 20 percent [from 186 to 223 pounds]. In 1993, a paper presented at a national symposium found that the preceding equation was especially accurate for predicting a 1-RM bench press (r=.99).

This formula is only valid for predicting a 1-RM when the number of repetitions-to-fatigue is less than 10. It should also be noted that if the repetitions exceed about 10, then the test becomes less accurate for evaluating anaerobic endurance as well as for estimating a 1-RM. In fact, a study published in 1995 (involving 220 subjects) compared six different equations and found that this formula was the only one of the six in which the predicted bench press did not differ significantly from the actual bench press (r=.98) when 10 or fewer repetitions were completed. At any rate, a test of anaerobic endurance — though not a direct measure of pure maximal strength — is much safer than a 1-RM lift because it involves a submaximal load. (Because genetic factors — particularly predominant muscle-fiber type — play a major role in anaerobic endurance, the aforementioned equation isn't accurate for everyone. However, the formula is still very practical for much of the population.)

Finally, the purpose of predicting a 1-RM shouldn't be to compare the strength of one person to another. It's unfair to make strength comparisons between individuals because each person has a different genetic potential for achieving muscular strength. Predicting a 1-RM is much more meaningful and fair when an individual's performance is compared to his or her last performance — not to the performance of others.

7. Is the adage "No pain, no gain" really true?

To a degree, yes. The most critical factor in achieving optimal results from cross training is your level of intensity or effort. As an exercise or activity becomes more intense, it also becomes more uncomfortable . . . and more painful. The discomfort and pain are related to the high concentration of blood lactic acid. (The effects of lactic acid accumulation are described in Chapter 3.) However, you must differentiate between muscular pain and orthopedic pain. Pain throughout a muscle during intense activity is normal and indicates a high degree of effort. Pain throughout a joint during intense activity is abnormal and indicates a possible orthopedic problem.

8. How do I know if I'm overtraining?

Overtraining is a result of overstressing the body. Generally, excessive stress is produced by performing excessive activity. Symptoms of overtraining include chronic fatigue, appetite disorders, insomnia, depression, anger, substantial weight loss or gain, muscle soreness, anemia and an elevated resting heart rate.

The most obvious indicator of overtraining, however, is a lack of progress in your muscular strength and/or aerobic fitness. A lack of progress can be identified by keeping accurate records of your performance. The best cure for overtraining is to obtain sufficient rest in order to allow your body the opportunity to recover. This may necessitate reducing the volume of activity that you perform. Taking some time off periodically from your cross-training activities also helps avoid overtraining.

9. What precautions should I take when cross training in hot, humid conditions?

The importance of safeguarding your body against heat-related injuries cannot be overemphasized. Overweight individuals and those who are unaccustomed to laboring in the heat are most susceptible to thermal disorders which include heat exhaustion, heat stroke and heat cramps.

 Under resting conditions, your core temperature is about 98.6 degrees Fahrenheit (or 37 degrees Celsius) and there is a balance between heat production and heat loss. During exercise, your core temperature increases and triggers several heat-loss mechanisms. The primary mechanism for heat loss during exercise is the evaporation of sweat. Your blood carries internal body heat to the surface of your skin where sweat is secreted from an estimated 2.5 million sweat glands and evaporation takes place. As the sweat evaporates it cools your skin; this in turn cools your blood. The cooled blood then returns to the warmer core and the cycle is repeated. This physiological process cools your internal body. (To illustrate the effects of evaporation, wet your finger and blow on it. You'll quickly note a cooling sensation as the evaporative process withdraws heat from your skin.)

It's hard to believe, but people are constantly perspiring. In cool, dry weather a relatively small amount of sweat is produced and the rate of evaporation can keep up with the rate of perspiration. In this case, your skin is dry to the touch and you aren't aware you're sweating — even though this alone may involve about a quart of water per day.

Unfortunately, this cooling mechanism doesn't work well when the heat or humidity is high. When the humidity is high, there's a lot of moisture already in the air. At higher levels of humidity, the evaporation of your sweat is hindered because the air is virtually saturated with water vapor and, as a result, there's no place for the extra moisture to go. This situation causes the body to overheat and may result in a heat-related injury. In fact, a temperature of only 80 degrees Fahrenheit becomes dangerous if the humidity reaches 90 percent.

You should gradually acclimatize to heat and humidity. This may necessitate initially performing outdoor cross-training activities during the cooler parts of the day such as the early morning and late evening. You should also adjust the length of your rest intervals according to the environmental conditions. Most adverse reactions to heat and humidity occur during the first few days of exercising outdoors. As you adapt to hot, humid conditions, you'll be able to exercise at greater levels of intensity while maintaining safe body temperatures. Another option is to move your cross-training activities indoors to air-conditioned surroundings — assuming, of course, that you have access to such an environment.

It's important for you to rehydrate with cold liquids as needed. You should measure your bodyweight each day before and after a cross-training session. In this way, you can monitor your water loss to determine if adequate rehydration is taking place. You should consume about 16 ounces of water for every pound of weight that you lose during exercise. Coaches who deny liquids to their athletes under adverse conditions are putting them at risk for a heat disorder.

To promote heat loss, you should wear clothing that is lightweight, light-colored and loose fitting. (Lighter colors reflect the sun's rays; darker colors absorb them.) Under no circumstances should you perform your cross-training activities in rubberized clothing or a "sauna suit." Exercising with the body covered in this manner can be lethal since these garments trap perspiration and cause the body to overheat rapidly.

10. When I exercise, why do I sometimes wheeze and cough and have a shortness of breath?

It has been estimated that as many as 80-percent of asthmatic people experience a condition known as "exercise-induced asthma" (EIA). As the name suggests, EIA is initiated by exercise. This condition can occur within the first handful of minutes of activity or a few hours following activity. Several factors contribute to EIA including the temperature and the humidity of the air you inhale. Breathing cold, dry air while exercising increases the likelihood of EIA. Certain intensities and durations of activity also contribute to EIA: The attacks are more likely during intense efforts of relatively long duration.

Anyone who suffers from EIA should seek the advice of a physician (who may prescribe medication as a preventive measure). If you must exercise outdoors in cold weather, you should cover your mouth with a scarf or face mask. Swimming is an excellent cross-training activity for those with EIA because the air above the pool is warm and contains moisture. Finally, those suffering from EIA should adjust their levels of intensity and the duration of their efforts accordingly.

11. Is it okay for me to perform sit-ups and leg lifts with my legs straight?

No. Sit-ups and leg lifts should never be performed with straight legs. Laying flat on your back with your hips and legs in an extended position exaggerates the arch in your low-back area. When your legs are extended, your iliopsoas muscle located on your frontal hip area is stretched and it tugs your lumbar spine into an exaggerated curve known as "lordosis." This position creates maximal peak compressive and shear forces in the lumbar region. On the other hand, when your knees and hips are bent and supported, your iliopsoas muscle is relaxed. This flattens your lumbar curvature and decreases the spinal load. Research using computer simulation has shown that compressive forces and shear forces are dramatically reduced during the performance of a sit-up exercise with the hips and the knees flexed at 90 degrees. When your hips and knees are in this position, your iliopsoas generates the least amount of tension. In brief, the compressive and shear forces in your lumbar region are minimized as the degree of hip flexion is maximized.

Your abdominals are used primarily during the first 30 degrees of a sit-up. Thereafter, your hip flexors accept most of the workload. For this reason, a partial sit-up — typically referred to as a "crunch" or a "trunk curl" in weight-room jargon — can be more effective than a full sit-up. This limited-range movement targets your abdominals and reduces the involvement of your hip flexors. It should also be noted that abdominal activity is greater when your feet are not held or fixed. (Stabilizing the feet activates the iliopsoas.)

To perform a trunk curl, lay on the floor and place the backs of your lower legs on a bench or a stool. The angle between your upper and lower legs should be about 90 degrees. Likewise, the angle between your upper legs and your torso should be about 90 degrees. Fold your arms across your chest and tuck your chin in to your torso so that your head is off the floor. Tucking your chin helps you to maintain a flat lower back throughout the movement, thereby reducing the amount of stress placed on your lumbar region during the performance of the exercise. To perform the movement, bring your torso up to your legs without snapping your head forward, pause briefly in this position and then return your torso back to the starting position. Your next repetition should be performed immediately after the bottom portions of your shoulder blades touch the floor. To maintain tension on your muscles throughout the sit-up movement, your upper shoulders should not contact the floor between repetitions.

Sit-ups — or any other exercise — should not be performed in a rapid, ballistic manner. Explosive movements create momentum which removes the workload from your muscles and makes the exercise less efficient. In the case of sit-ups, rapid flexion of your spine can place excessive stress on the posterior structures of your lumbar area and may ultimately lead to its degeneration.

Performing leg lifts with straight legs does little to activate your abdominal muscles. Rather, the iliopsoas muscle is most active and tends to pull your lumbar spine into lordosis. Because of this, knee-ups should be performed instead of leg lifts with straight legs. To do knee-ups, simply hang from a chinning bar or support yourself between two dip handles and pull your knees up to your chest. Under no circumstances should you do "Roman Chair" sit-ups. This particular movement hyperextends the spine and places undue stress on the low-back area which has led to numerous injuries.

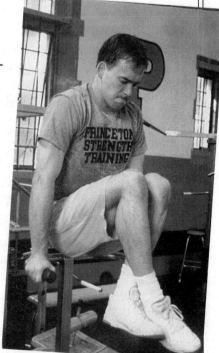

12. Wouldn't I get better results by strength training different body parts on alternate days instead of doing all of them on one day?

Not necessarily. Exercising different body parts on alternating days is known as a "split routine." This has been a popular training method of bodybuilders and recreational lifters for

Right: Knee-ups (pictured) should be performed instead of leg lifts with straight legs. (Photo by Matt Brzycki)

many years. In this type of routine, a person works out on consecutive days but exercises different muscles. For example, the muscle groups might be "split" such that the lower body is exercised on Mondays and Thursdays and the upper body is trained on Tuesdays and Fridays.

It's certainly true that a person who uses a split routine doesn't usually exercise the same muscles two days in a row. Recall, however, that it takes a minimum of 48 hours in order for your body to replenish its stockpiles of carbohydrates following an intense workout. (Again, carbohydrates are the principal fuel during intense exercise.) So, if you exercised your lower body intensely on Monday, your carbohydrate stores were severely depleted. Even if you involve different muscles on Tuesday, your body hasn't had the necessary 48 hours to fully recover those carbohydrate stores.

From an athletic perspective, split routines aren't recommended because they aren't specific to the muscular involvement of any sport or activity. When you use a split routine, you exercise different muscles on different days. However, a selective use of your muscles never happens in an athletic competition. In virtually any sport or activity, athletes are required to integrate all of their muscle groups at once. Therefore, it makes little sense for athletes to prepare for competition by training their muscles separately on different days.

There are individual variations in recovery ability, but split routines are generally inappropriate, inefficient and unreasonable for the majority of the population. Remember, the most efficient program is one that gives you the maximum possible results in the least amount of time.

13. Are Strength Shoes good for increasing my speed, quickness and explosive power?

Not according to several studies. The Strength Shoe is a modified athletic shoe with a four-centimeter thick rubber platform attached to the front half of the sole. This attachment prevents your heel from striking the ground during exercises and drills. The shoe is touted as an effective method of increasing ankle flexibility, calf circumference and "speed, quickness and explosive power" when used in a plyometric-based training protocol. (Question 16 of this chapter discusses plyometrics in greater detail.)

A study published in 1993 found that subjects who performed a 10-minute jump-training program in Strength Shoes (or regular athletic shoes for that matter) did not significantly increase their vertical-jump height greater than the subjects who acted as controls.

Another 1993 study reported no enhancement of flexibility, strength or performance for participants wearing the Strength Shoe at the end of an 8-week training program — despite following the suggested protocol of the manufacturers. In this particular study, it's important to note that one third of the subjects who wore the Strength Shoes complained of anterior tibial pain (i.e., shin splints) and one subject withdrew from the study because the pain was severe. All of the subjects were previously involved in strenuous activities and none of the subjects reported leg pain prior to the study. Additionally, no subject who wore normal training shoes reported leg pain. As such, the authors felt that "the pain was device-related." In summation, the researchers concluded, "The use of the Strength Shoe cannot be recommended as a safe, effective training method for development of lower-leg strength and flexibility."

14. Isn't low-intensity exercise more effective for fat loss than high-intensity exercise?

Not really. A greater percentage of carbohydrates are used as an energy source during exercise of higher intensity. Conversely, a greater percentage of fats are used as an energy source during exercise of lower intensity. (Carbohydrates are a more efficient source of energy. However, fats are used as an energy source because your body doesn't need to be efficient at lower levels of intensity.) These physiological facts have led to the mistaken belief that "fat-burning" (or low-intensity) exercise is better than "carbohydrate-burning" (or high-intensity) exercise when it comes to losing weight, "burning" fat and expending calories. Unfortunately, this misconception continues to be endorsed by many fitness professionals and has spawned the hyped-up notion of a "fat-burning zone."

The concept of keeping the exercise intensity low in order to mobilize and selectively utilize a higher percentage of fat may sound logical, but it doesn't hold up mathematically and has never been verified in the laboratory. In truth, even though the percentage of calories used from fats are greater during low-intensity exercise, the total number of calories expended during high-intensity exercise is greater.

During any activity, your rate of caloric expenditure is directly related to your intensity of effort — the higher your intensity, the greater the rate of caloric expenditure. In the case of running, for example, your intensity is directly associated with your speed — the faster you run, the greater the rate of caloric utilization. The time of your activity is also a factor — the longer that you perform a given activity, the greater the total caloric expenditure.

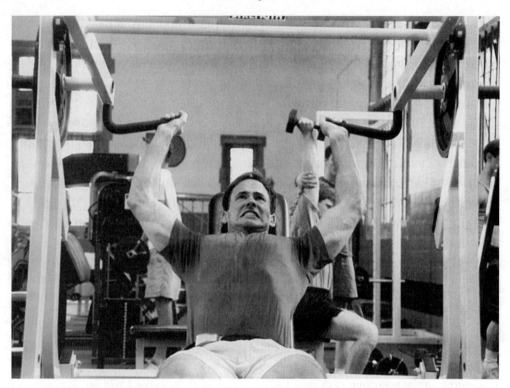

Based upon scientific equations for determining oxygen intake and caloric expenditure during walking and running, a 165-pound man who walks 3 miles in 60 minutes will utilize roughly 4.33 calories per minute (cal/min). Over the course of his 60-minute walk, his total caloric usage would be about 260 calories [4.33 cal/min x 60 min]. If that same individual ran those 3 miles in 30 minutes, he would use about 13.38 cal/min. (Note the higher rate of caloric utilization.) During his 30-minute effort, he would have expended about 401 total calories [13.38 cal/min x 30 min]. So, exercising at a higher level of intensity used up significantly more calories than exercising at a lower level of intensity [401 cal compared to 260 cal]. This is true despite the fact that the activity of lower intensity was performed for twice as long as the activity of higher intensity. (Chapter 4 offers formulas for determining oxygen intake and caloric expenditure during walking and running.)

These calculations have been corroborated by research performed in the laboratory. In one study, a group of subjects walked on a treadmill at an average speed of 3.8 miles per hour (mph) for 30 minutes. In this instance, the subjects used an average of about 8 cal/min for a total caloric expenditure of 240 calories [8 cal/min x 30 min]. Of these 240 calories, 59 percent

Above: Low-intensity exercise is not more effective for fat loss than high-intensity exercise. (Photo by Matt Brzycki)

[144 cal] were from carbohydrates and 41 percent [96 cal] were from fats. As part of the study, the same group also ran on a treadmill at an average speed of 6.5 mph for 30 minutes. At this relatively higher level of intensity, the subjects used an average of about 15 cal/min for a total caloric expenditure of 450 calories [15 cal/min x 30 min]. Of these 450 calories, 76 percent [342 cal] were from carbohydrates and 24 percent [108 cal] were from fats. In other words, exercising at a higher level of intensity resulted in a greater total caloric expenditure than exercising at a lower level of intensity [450 cal versus 240 cal] and also used a greater number of calories from fats in the same length of time [108 cal compared to 96 cal]. Additional studies have also demonstrated that more calories are expended when running a given distance than walking the same distance.

The intent behind advocating low-intensity exercise of long duration is to enhance safety and improve compliance in the non-athletic population. However, low-intensity exercise is not more effective for fat loss than high-intensity exercise. In order to lose weight, more calories must be expended than consumed to produce a caloric deficit. Whether carbohydrates or fats are used to produce this caloric shortfall is immaterial. A caloric deficit created by the selective use of fat as an energy source doesn't necessarily translate into greater fat loss compared to an equal caloric deficit created by the use of carbohydrate as an energy source.

In short, researchers who perform studies and review the scientific literature in the area of exercise and weight control generally agree that it probably doesn't matter whether you use fats or carbohydrates while exercising in order to lose weight. Finally, it should also be noted that low-intensity exercise usually doesn't elevate the heart rate enough in healthy adults to produce an aerobic cross-training effect. (Chapter 9 discusses the subject of weight loss in greater detail.)

15. Why are my muscles no longer sore the day after I work out?

There are two types of muscle soreness: acute and delayed-onset. Acute muscle soreness occurs during and immediately following exercise. One theory suggests that this soreness is associated with an occlusion of blood flow to your muscles (ischemia). Because of the lack of adequate blood flow, metabolic waste products (e.g., lactic acid) cannot be removed and accumulate to the point of stimulating the pain receptors in your muscles. On the other hand, delayed-onset muscular soreness (DOMS) refers to the pain and soreness that occurs 24 - 48 hours after exercise. The exact cause of DOMS is unknown. The most popular theory is that cellular damage occurs to the muscle fibers and/or connective tissue such as tendons.

Just because you don't experience DOMS the day after a workout doesn't mean your efforts weren't effective. If you accidentally bumped your shin, your lower-leg area may be sore next day — and perhaps for a few days afterwards. However, this doesn't mean the soreness was productive.

So, muscle soreness — or lack thereof — isn't necessarily an indicator of your efforts. DOMS can result from several situations. You'll experience DOMS if you've done an excessive amount of exercise. In this case, the soreness doesn't mean your workout was productive. Excessive maybe, but not necessarily productive. You'll also probably get sore if you do something unfamiliar in your workout such as changing your order of exercises, your equipment (e.g., using free weights instead of a machine or vice versa) or your exercises (e.g., doing a pressing movement while laying on an incline bench instead of a flat bench). In all likelihood, you'll also encounter DOMS if you increase your level of intensity or take less recovery time than usual between your exercises.

But again, just because your muscles aren't sore the next day doesn't mean your workout wasn't productive . . . or that you didn't do enough sets or exercises. Similarly, having muscular soreness following a workout doesn't mean that it was productive — it could simply indicate that you did something that was unfamiliar.

For those concerned with becoming sore, your potential for DOMS is reduced as you grow accustomed to the specific demands of an activity. A gradual progression in your intensity also helps reduce the possibility of excessive muscular soreness.

16. Will plyometrics improve my vertical jump?

Not necessarily. The term "plyometrics" applies to any exercise or jumping drill that uses the myotatic or stretch reflex of a muscle. This particular reflex is triggered when a muscle is pre-stretched prior to a muscular contraction, resulting in a more powerful movement than would otherwise be possible. For example, just before jumping vertically — such as for a rebound — you bend at your hips and knees. This "countermovement" pre-stretches your hip and leg muscles allowing you to generate more force than if you performed the jump without first squatting down. Popular exercises based on this principle include bounding, hopping and various box drills (such as depth jumping). Upper-body plyometrics frequently incorporate medicine balls to induce the myotatic reflex.

Plyometrics are highly controversial. Most of the support for plyometrics is based upon personal narratives and sketchy research. There is little scientific evidence that definitively proves plyometrics are productive. While muscular force is certainly increased by the pre-stretch mechanism, it doesn't necessarily follow that a training adaptation occurs. In reality, a large number of research studies have concluded that plyometrics are no more effective than regular strength-training activities when it comes to improving leg strength, jumping ability, speed and power. One plyometric guru even admits that the information about plyometrics is anecdotal and "methodologically weak."

More importantly, the possibility of injury from plyometrics is positively enormous. A growing number of strength and fitness professionals are questioning the safety of plyometrics. When performing plyometrics, the musculoskeletal system is exposed to repetitive trauma and high-impact forces. This extreme biomechanical loading places an inordinate amount of strain on the connective tissues of the lower body. The most common plyometric-related injuries are patellar tendinitis, stress fractures, shin splints and strains of the ankle and the knee. Compression fractures related to the use of plyometrics have also been reported. Other potential injuries include — but aren't limited to — sprains, heel bruises, ruptured tendons and meniscal (cartilage) damage. Youths are especially vulnerable. It's no surprise that many prominent orthopedic surgeons, physical therapists and athletic trainers view plyometrics as an injury waiting to happen.

Further research is needed to determine if plyometric exercises are safe and effective. At this point in time, plyometrics have not been proven to be productive and carry an unreasonably high risk of injury. You can improve your vertical jump in a much safer manner by simply practicing your jumping skills and techniques in the same way that they are used in your sport or activity and by strengthening your major muscle groups, especially your hips and legs.

17. Won't lifting weights make females less flexible and bulk them up?

No. One of the biggest misconceptions in strength training is the belief that females who lift weights will lose flexibility and develop large, unsightly muscles. It was noted in Chapter 6 that a properly conducted strength-training program does not reduce flexibility. Exercising throughout a full range of motion against a resistance maintains or even improves flexibility. Females who have residual fears about becoming less flexible can perform a comprehensive stretching routine both before and after their strength-training program. As an added measure, the muscles can also be stretched immediately following the completion of each exercise. (See Chapter 8 for more information on stretching.)

Since the early 1960s, research has demonstrated that females can achieve significant improvements in muscular strength without concomitant gains in muscle size. For instance, a study published in 1974 found that the largest increase in muscle size experienced by any of the 47 females in the study was less than one-quarter inch. Clearly, strength training does not lead to excessive muscular bulk or produce masculinizing effects in the majority of females.

There are several physiological reasons that prevent or minimize the possibility of a female significantly increasing the size of her muscles. First of all, most females are genetically bound by an unfavorable and unchangeable ratio of muscle to tendon (i.e., short muscle bellies coupled with long tendinous attachments). In addition, compared to males most females have low levels of serum testosterone. The low level of this growth-promoting hormone restricts the degree of muscular hypertrophy in females.

A final physiological factor that prevents or minimizes the possibility of a female significantly increasing her muscular size is her percentage of body fat. Quite simply, females tend to inherit higher percentages of body fat than do males. For example, the average 18- to 22-year-old female is about 22 - 26 percent body fat, whereas the average male of similar age is about 12 - 16 percent. The higher the percentage of body fat, the lower the percentage of muscle mass. This extra body fat also tends to soften or mask the effects of strength training. Females who possess very little subcutaneous body fat appear more muscular than they actually are because their muscles are more visible. Similarly, the appearance of muscle mass following a strength-training program may not be the result of muscular hypertrophy. Rather, a decrease in

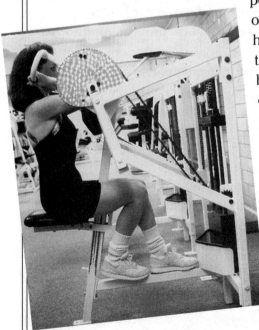

Left: It's physiologically improbable for the average female to develop large muscles that are unsightly or unfeminine. (Photo by Matt Brzycki)

subcutaneous fat may simply make the same amount of muscle mass become more noticeable.

In the case of female bodybuilders, they inherit a greater potential for muscular hypertrophy than the average female. Highly competitive female bodybuilders have developed large muscles because of their genetic potential — not because they were engaged in bodybuilding activities.

There is a relatively small number of females who have inherited the ingredients necessary to experience significant muscular hypertrophy from strength training. However, the majority of females can gain considerable strength from a strength-training program yet have little or no change in their muscle mass. In short, it's physiologically improbable for the average female to develop large muscles that are unsightly or unfeminine.

18. Can I do anything to increase the intensity of an exercise after I reach muscular fatigue?

Yes. After you've reached concentric muscular fatigue, you can increase your intensity by immediately performing several additional intensification (or post-fatigue) repetitions.

One popular intensification technique is the use of "negatives." Recall from Chapter 2 that raising a weight is sometimes referred to as the positive phase of a movement and involves a concentric muscular contraction; lowering a weight is typically referred to as the negative phase of a movement and involves an eccentric muscular contraction. Your eccentric strength is always greater than your concentric (and isometric) strength. This means that when you reach a point where you are unable to raise a weight concentrically, you still have the ability to lower the weight eccentrically. Herein lies the reasoning and the value behind performing negatives after reaching concentric muscle fatigue at the end of a set. In a negative repetition, your training partner raises the weight concentrically while you (the lifter) lower the weight eccentrically. This is repeated for 3 - 5 repetitions with each repetition lasting about 6 - 8 seconds (depending upon the range of motion).

As an example, suppose that you reached concentric muscular fatigue on a barbell bench press. Your partner would help you raise the weight off your chest until your arms are extended. Then, you lower the weight under control back to your chest. Your partner can even add a little extra resistance by pushing down on the bar as you lower it. These are called "forced reps." In effect, these post-fatigue repetitions are positive-assisted and negative-resisted.

Performing a few negative repetitions at the end of an exercise allows you to reach eccentric muscular fatigue — when your muscles have fatigued to the point that you can't even lower the weight. And that's why a set-to-fatigue followed immediately by several negatives is so brutally effective: You've managed to exhaust your muscles completely — both concentrically and eccentrically.

Another popular intensification technique is the use of "regressions" which are also called "breakdowns" or "burnouts." When performing regressions, you (or your training partner) quickly reduce the starting weight by about 25 - 30 percent and you (the lifter) do 3 - 5 regression repetitions with the lighter resistance. Let's say you just did 14 repetitions with 100 pounds on the leg extension and reached concentric muscular fatigue. You (or your training partner) would immediately reduce the weight to about 70 - 75 pounds and would then attempt to perform 3 - 5 repetitions with the lighter weight.

If you desire, you can do a second "series" of regressions. Using the previous example, you'd immediately reduce the 70 - 75 pounds to about 50 - 55 pounds and attempt to perform 3 - 5 repetitions with that weight.

Remember, it all comes down to producing a sufficient level of muscle fatigue. If you don't create enough muscle fatigue then you did little to stimulate gains in your muscular size and strength. On the other hand, if you create too much muscle fatigue then you may also experience submaximal gains in muscle size and strength. Therefore, these two types of intensification repetitions should be used sparingly.

19. Isn't it true that lifting weights explosively will increase speed, power and quickness?

No! Lifting weights at rapid speeds of movement is only a demonstration of power — not an adaptation. There's absolutely no scientific evidence to suggest that "explosive" lifting leads to "explosive" athletic performance.

High-velocity movements are actually less productive than movements performed in a slow, deliberate manner. Here's why: Whenever a weight is lifted explosively, momentum is introduced to provide movement to the weight or resistance. After the initial explosive movement, little or no resistance is encountered by the muscles throughout the remaining range of motion. In simple terms, the weight is practically moving under its own power. To illustrate the effects of momentum on muscular tension, imagine that you pushed a 100-pound cart across the length of a basketball court at a deliberate, steady pace. In this instance, you applied a constant load to your muscles for the entire distance. Now, suppose that you were to push the cart across the court again. This time, however, you accelerated your pace to the point where you were running as fast as possible. If you were to stop pushing the cart at mid-court, it would continue to move by itself because you gave it momentum. So, in this case, your muscles had resistance over the first half of the court . . . but not over the last half of the court. The same effect occurs in the weight room. When weights are lifted explosively, there is a load on your muscles over the initial part of the movement . . . but not over the last part. In effect, the requirement for muscular force is reduced and so are the potential strength gains.

Unfortunately, the limited effects due to the use of momentum are demonstrated in weight rooms across the world on a daily basis — albeit, in most cases, unknowingly. For example, have you ever raised a weight so quickly on a leg extension machine that the pad left your lower legs halfway through the repetition? Well, the pad is attached to the movement arm of the machine which, in turn, is connected to the resistance by some means — such as a chain, cable or strap. If the pad is no longer in contact with your lower legs, there's no load on your muscles. If there's no load on your muscles, then your muscles have no stimulus — or reason — to adapt. Sure, your muscles were "loaded" during the first part of the movement — while the pad was still against your shins — and you'll get some results from the exercise. But during the last part of the movement — when the pad left your shins — you won't get any results. At that point, the only load or resistance your muscles encounter is from the weight of your lower legs. There's no question that momentum makes an exercise less efficient and less productive.

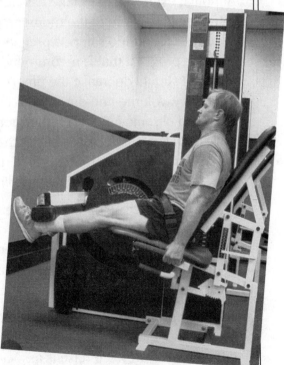

Explosive lifting can also be dangerous. If explosive lifting doesn't cause immediate musculoskeletal damage, it will certainly predispose you to

Right: It's much safer and more efficient to raise the weight without any jerking or explosive movements and to lower it under control. (Photo by Matt Brzycki)

future injury. Dr. Fred Allman, a past president of the American College of Sports Medicine, states, "It is even possible that many injuries . . . may be the result of weakened connective tissue caused by explosive training in the weight room." Using momentum to lift a weight increases the internal forces encountered by a given joint; the faster a weight is lifted, the greater these forces are amplified — especially at the point of explosion. When the forces exceed the structural limits of a joint, an injury occurs in the muscles, bones or connective tissue.

It's much safer and more efficient to raise the weight without any jerking or explosive movements and to lower it under control. Raising the weight in about 1 - 2 seconds and lowering it in about 3 - 4 seconds ensures that the speed of movement is not ballistic in nature and that momentum does not play a significant role in the efficiency of the exercise.

20. Should I exercise during my pregnancy?

Proper exercise — including strength training — poses little risk to either the mother or the developing fetus. However, women who have never partici-pated in an exercise program should not begin one during their pregnancy. Regardless, you should consult your physician before you initiate any exer-cise program.

Although exercise poses little risk during pregnancy, there is the potential for adverse effects to both the mother and the fetus. With several precautionary measures for added safety, a pregnant female can perform the same type of exercise program that is recommended for the general population. In gen-eral, you should decrease the program variables — such as the intensity, frequency, volume and duration — if you exhibit signs of exertional intoler-ance and chronic fatigue. Furthermore, you should immediately consult your physician if you experience any of the following warning signs or complica-tions: abdominal pain or cramping, ruptured membranes, elevated blood pressure or heart rate, vaginal bleeding or a lack of fetal movement.

When you exercise, there is an increased blood flow to your working skel-etal muscles. During pregnancy, the diversion of oxygen-rich blood to your exercising muscles leads to a transient reduction in blood flow and oxygen to the fetus. However, low- to moderate-intensity exercise of less than 30 minutes does not seem to disturb uterine blood flow.

Another concern for the developing fetus — especially during the first tri-mester of pregnancy — is exercise-induced hyperthermia (i.e., an increased core temperature). Exercise is associated with a rise in both maternal and fetal body core temperature. In order to dissipate heat, the fetus must depend entirely on your thermoregulatory abilities. To avoid heat complications, you must be adequately hydrated, exercise at a level of intensity that is lower than your pre-pregnancy state and wear light clothing that permits heat loss. In addition, you must be aware of the existing environmental temperature and humidity. During pregnancy, women should not exercise when the ambient temperature is greater than 90 degrees Fahrenheit and the relative humidity exceeds 50 percent. Finally, an exercise program should not exceed 30 minutes in duration so as not to expose the fetus to prolonged thermal stress.

Pregnancy increases the laxity of your ligaments and joints. This allows your ribs and pelvic cavity to expand in order to encompass your growing baby and make delivery easier. However, connective tissue softens throughout your entire body and your joints become less stable. The increased joint and connective tissue laxity may make you more susceptible to low-back, hip, knee and ankle injuries during pregnancy.

When strength training, you should use slightly higher repetition ranges than suggested for the general population. The higher repetition ranges require the use of lighter resistance, which reduces the orthopedic stress placed upon your vulnerable joint structures. Additionally, you shouldn't overstretch or perform exercises in a ballistic manner. The aim of flexibility programs during pregnancy should be to relieve muscle cramping or soreness and relax your lower-back region to alleviate pain. Weightbearing, high-impact activities — such as running, jumping, hopping and bouncing — should be eliminated, minimized or replaced with low-impact, non-weightbearing ones.

According to the American College of Obstetricians and Gynecologists, you shouldn't perform exercise in the supine (laying face-up) position after the fourth month of your pregnancy. When in the supine position, the excess weight of the enlarging fetus may obstruct the flow of blood back to your heart.

Your intake of calories must be sufficient to meet the extra energy needs of pregnancy and any activities that you performed. During pregnancy, you need to consume about 300 additional calories per day (not counting the additional caloric requirements of any activities you do).

References

American College of Sports Medicine [ACSM]. 1990. Position statement on the recommended quantity and quality of exercise for developing and maintaining cardiorespiratory and muscular fitness in healthy adults. *Medicine and Science in Sports and Exercise* 22: 265-274.

_____. 1991. *Guidelines for graded exercise testing and exercise prescription.* 4th ed. Philadelphia: Lea & Febiger.

American Council on Exercise [ACE]. 1991. *Personal trainer manual: The resource for fitness instructors.* San Diego: ACE.

American Dietetic Association [ADA]. 1987. Position of the ADA: Nutrition for physical fitness and athletic performance for adults. *Journal of the American Dietetic Association* 87 (7): 933-939.

Asimov, I. 1992. *The human body: Its structure and operation.* Revised ed. New York: Mentor.

Astrand, I. 1960. Aerobic work capacity in men and women with special reference to age. *Acta Physiologica Scandinavica* 49 (Supplementum 169): 1-92.

Astrand, P.O., and K. Rodahl. 1977. *Textbook of work physiology.* 2d ed. New York: McGraw-Hill Book Company.

Bates, B., M. Wolf and J. Blunk. 1990. *Vanderbilt university strength and conditioning manual.* Nashville, TN: Vanderbilt University.

Ben-Ezra, V. 1992. Assessing physical fitness. In *The Stairmaster fitness handbook*, ed. J. A. Peterson and C. X. Bryant, 91-108. Indianapolis: Masters Press.

Brown, C. H., and J. H. Wilmore. 1974. The effects of maximal resistance training on the strength and body composition of women athletes. *Medicine and Science in Sports and Exercise* 6: 174-177.

Bryant, C. X. 1995. Understanding crossrobic training. In *The Stairmaster fitness handbook*, 2d ed, ed. J. A. Peterson and C. X. Bryant, 81-105. St. Louis: Wellness Bookshelf.

Bryant, C. X., and J. A. Peterson. 1992. Estimating aerobic fitness. *Fitness Management* 9 (August): 36-39.

Bryant, C. X., and J. A. Peterson. 1993. Active pregnancy. *Fitness Management* 10 (October): 36-37, 40-42.

Bryant, C. X., and J. A. Peterson. 1994. Strength training for the heart? *Fitness Management* 10 (February): 32-34.

Bryant, C. X., J. A. Peterson and R. J. Hagen. 1994. Weight loss: Unfolding the truth. *Fitness Management* 10 (May): 42-44.

Bryant, C. X., and J. A. Peterson. 1996. All exercise is not equal. *Fitness Management* 12 (July): 32-34.

Brzycki, M. M. 1995. *A practical approach to strength training*. 3d ed. Indianapolis: Masters Press.

_____. 1995. *Youth strength and conditioning*. Indianapolis: Masters Press.

_____. 1993. Strength testing — predicting a one-rep max from reps-to-fatigue. *The Journal of Physical Education, Recreation & Dance* 64 (1): 88-90.

Brzycki, M. M., and S. Brown. 1993. *Conditioning for basketball*. Indianapolis: Masters Press.

Bubb, W. J. 1992. Nutrition. In *Health fitness instructor's handbook*, 2d ed, by E. T. Howley and B. D. Franks, 95-114. Champaign, IL: Human Kinetics Publishers, Inc.

City of New York Department of Consumer Affairs. 1992. *Magic muscle pills!! Health and fitness quackery in nutrition supplements*. New York, NY: Department of Consumer Affairs.

Clark, N. 1990. *Nancy Clark's sports nutrition guidebook*. Champaign, IL: Leisure Press.

Clausen, J. P. 1977. Effect of training on cardiovascular adjustments to exercise in man. *Physiological Reviews* 57: 779-815.

Cook, S. D., G. Schultz, M. L. Omey, M. W. Wolfe and M. F. Brunet. 1993. Development of lower leg strength and flexibility with the strength shoe. *The American Journal of Sports Medicine* 21: 445-448.

Costill, D. L., J. Daniels, W. Evans, W. F. Fink, G. S. Krahenbuhl and B. Saltin. 1976. Skeletal muscle enzymes and fiber composition in male and female track athletes. *Journal of Applied Physiology* 40: 149-154.

Cress, M. A., and D. Colacino. 1992. Developing exercise prescriptions for older adults. In *The Stairmaster fitness handbook*, ed. J. A. Peterson and C. X. Bryant, 137-150. Indianapolis: Masters Press.

Crouch, J. E. 1978. *Functional human anatomy.* 3d ed. Philadelphia: Lea & Febiger.

Daniels, J. 1989. *Training distance runners — a primer.* Sports Science Exchange 1 (11): 1-4.

Desmedt, J. E., and E. Godaux. 1977. Fast motor units are not preferentially activated in rapid voluntary contractions in man. *Nature* 267: 717-719.

deVries, H. A. 1974. *Physiology of exercise for physical education and athletics.* 2d ed. Dubuque, IA: William C. Brown.

Dintiman, G. B. 1984. *How to run faster.* West Point, NY: Leisure Press.

Dunn, J. R. 1989. Developing strength the L. A. Raiders way. *Strength and Fitness Quarterly* 1 (1): 7.

Enoka, R. M. 1988. *Neuromechanical basis of kinesiology.* Champaign, IL: Human Kinetics Publishers, Inc.

_____. 1988. Muscle strength and its development. *Sports Medicine* 6: 146-168.

Farley, D. 1993. Dietary supplements: Making sure hype doesn't overwhelm science. *FDA Consumer* 27 (November): 8-13.

Fellingham, G. W., E. S. Roundy, A. G. Fisher and G. R. Bryce. 1978. Caloric cost of walking and running. *Medicine and Science in Sports and Exercise* 10: 132-136.

Ferrando, A., and N. Green. 1993. The effect of boron supplementation on lean body mass, plasma testosterone levels and strength in bodybuilders. *International Journal of Sports Nutrition* 3 (2): 140-149.

Fink, K. J., and B. Worthington-Roberts. 1995. Nutritional considerations for exercise. In *The Stairmaster fitness handbook*, 2d ed, ed. J. A. Peterson and C. X. Bryant, 205-228. St. Louis: Wellness Bookshelf.

Fox, E. L., and D. K. Mathews. 1981. *The physiological basis of physical education and athletics*. 3d ed. Philadelphia: Saunders College Publishing.

Fox, E. L. 1984. Physiology of exercise and physical fitness. In *Sports medicine*, ed. R. H. Strauss, 381-456. Philadelphia: W. B. Saunders Company.

Frankel, V. H., and M. Nordin. 1980. *Basic biomechanics of the skeletal system*. Philadelphia: Lea & Febiger.

Garrett Jr, W. E., and T. R. Malone, eds. 1988. *Muscle development: Nutritional alternatives to anabolic steroids*. Columbus, OH: Ross Laboratories.

Gettman, L. R., P. Ward and R. D. Hagman. 1982. A comparison of combined running and weight training with circuit weight training. *Medicine and Science in Sports and Exercise* 14: 229-234.

Gittleson, M. 1984. *Michigan football off-season conditioning*. Ann Arbor, MI: University of Michigan.

Goldberg, A. L., J. D. Etlinger, D. F. Goldspink and C. Jablecki. 1975. Mechanism of work-induced hypertrophy of skeletal muscle. *Medicine and Science in Sports* 7: 248-261.

Graves, J. E., and M. L. Pollock. 1995. Understanding the physiological basis of muscular fitness. In *The Stairmaster fitness handbook*, 2d ed, ed. J. A. Peterson and C. X. Bryant, 67-80. St. Louis: Wellness Bookshelf.

Guthrie, H. A. 1983. *Introductory nutrition*. 5th ed. St. Louis: The C. V. Mosby Company.

Hakkinen, K., A. Pakarinen and M. Kallinen. 1992. Neuromuscular adaptations and serum hormones in women during short-term intensive strength training. *European Journal of Applied Physiology* 64: 106-111.

Hay, J. G., and J. G. Reid. 1988. *Anatomy, mechanics, and human motion*. 2d ed. Englewood Cliffs, NJ: Prentice-Hall, Inc.

Hellebrandt, F. A., and S. J. Houtz. 1956. Mechanisms of muscle training in man: Experimental demonstration of the overload principle. *Physical Therapy Review* 36: 371-383.

Hempel, L. S., and C. L. Wells. 1985. Cardiorespiratory cost of the Nautilus express circuit. *The Physician and Sportsmedicine* 13 (4): 86-86, 91-97.

Herbert, V., and G. J. Subak-Sharpe, eds. 1990. *The Mount Sinai school of medicine complete book of nutrition*. New York, NY: St. Martin's Press.

Hickson, R. C., C. Kanakis, J. R. Davis, A. M. Moore and S. Rich. 1982. Reduced training duration effects on aerobic power, endurance and cardiac growth. *Journal of Applied Physiology* 53: 225-229.

Hill, A. V. 1922. The maximum work and mechanical efficiency in human muscles, and their most economical speed. *Journal of Physiology* 56: 19-41.

Hoeger, W. W. K. 1988. *Principles and labs for physical fitness and wellness*. Englewood, CO: Morton Publishing Co.

Howley, E. T., and B. D. Franks. 1992. *Health fitness instructor's handbook*. 2d ed. Champaign, IL: Human Kinetics Publishers, Inc.

Howley, E. T., and M. Glover. 1974. The caloric costs of running and walking one mile for men and women. *Medicine and Science in Sports and Exercise* 6: 235-237.

Hurley, B. F., D. R. Seals, A. A. Ehsani, L.-J. Cartier, G. P. Dalsky, J. M. Hagberg and J. O. Holloszy. 1984. Effects of high-intensity strength training on cardiovascular function. *Medicine and Science in Sports and Exercise* 16: 483-488.

Hutchins, K. 1992. *Super Slow: The ultimate exercise protocol*. 2d ed. Casselberry, FL: Super Slow Systems.

Huxley, H. E. 1958. The contraction of muscle. *Scientific American* 199 (5): 66-82.

_____. 1965. The mechanism of muscular contraction. *Scientific American* 213 (6): 18-27.

Ivy, J. L. 1991. Muscle glycogen synthesis before and after exercise. *Sports Medicine* 11 (1): 6-19.

Johnson, C., and J. G. Reid. 1991. Lumbar compressive and shear forces during various trunk curl-up exercises. *Clinical Biomechanics* 6: 97-104.

Jones, A. 1970. *Nautilus training principles, bulletin #1*. DeLand, FL: Arthur Jones Productions.

_____. 1971. *Nautilus training principles, bulletin #2*. DeLand, FL: Arthur Jones Productions.

_____. 1993. *The lumbar spine, the cervical spine and the knee: Testing and rehabilitation.* Ocala, FL: MedX Corporation.

Jones, A., M. L. Pollock, J. E. Graves, M. Fulton, W. Jones, M. MacMillan. D. D. Baldwin and J. Cirulli. 1988. *Safe, specific testing and rehabilitative exercise of the muscles of the lumbar spine.* Santa Barbara, CA: Sequoia Communications.

Jones, N. L., N. McCartney and A. J. McComas, eds. 1986. *Human muscle power.* Champaign, IL: Human Kinetics Publishers, Inc.

Kalamen, J. 1968. Measurement of maximum muscle power in man. Doctoral dissertation. Columbus, OH: The Ohio State University.

Karlsson, J., P. V. Komi and J. H. T. Viitasalo. 1979. Muscle strength and muscle characteristics in monozygous and dizygous twins. *Acta Physiologica Scandinavica* 106: 319-325.

Kennedy, P. M. 1986. Setting the record straight about negative exercise. *Scholastic Coach* 56 (November): 22-23, 69.

Klissouras, V. 1971. Heritability of adaptive variation. *Journal of Applied Physiology* 31: 338-344.

Komi, P. V., J. H. T. Viitasalo, M. Havu, A. Thorstensson, B. Sjodin and J. Karlsson. 1977. Skeletal muscle fibers and muscle enzyme activities in monozygous and dizygous twins of both sexes. *Acta Physiologica Scandinavica* 100: 385-392.

Komi, P. V., and J. Karlsson. 1979. Physical performance, skeletal muscle enzyme activities and fiber types in monozygous and dizygous twins of both sexes. *Acta Physiologica Scandinavica* (Supplementum 462): 1-28.

Kraemer, W. J. 1992. Involvement of eccentric muscle action may optimize adaptations to resistance training. *Sports Science Exchange* 4 (6): 1-4.

Krahenbuhl, G. S., P. A. Archer and L. L. Pettit. 1978. Serum testosterone and adult female trainability. *Journal of Sports Medicine and Physical Fitness* 18: 359-364.

Kris-Etherton, P. M. 1989. The facts and fallacies of nutritional supplements for athletes. *Sports Science Exchange* 2 (8): 1-4.

Lamb, D. R. 1984. *Physiology of exercise: Responses & adaptations.* 2d ed. New York, NY: MacMillan Publishing Company.

Leistner, K. E. 1986. The quality repetition. *The Steel Tip 2* (June): 6-7.

_____. 1989. Explosive training: Not necessary. *High Intensity Training Newsletter 1* (2): 3-5.

Lesmes, G. R., D. W. Benham, D. L. Costill and W. J. Fink. 1983. Glycogen utilization in fast and slow twitch muscle fibers during maximal isokinetic exercise. *Annals of Sports Medicine* 1: 105-108.

LeSuer, D. A., and J. H. McCormick. 1993. Prediction of a 1-RM bench press and 1-RM squat from repetitions to fatigue using the Brzycki formula. Abstract presented at the National Strength and Conditioning Association 16th National Conference. Las Vegas, NV.

Lieber, D. C., R. L. Lieber and W. C. Adams. 1989. Effects of run-training and swim-training at similar absolute intensities on treadmill VO2 max. *Medicine and Science in Sports and Exercise* 21: 655-661.

Lillegard, W. A., and J. D. Terrio. 1994. Appropriate strength training. *Sports Medicine* 78: 457-477.

Londeree, B. R., and M. L. Moeschberger. 1982. Effect of age and other factors on maximal heart rate. *Research Quarterly for Exercise and Sport* 53: 297-304.

Lowenthal, D. T., and Y. Karni. 1990. The nutritional needs of athletes. In *The Mount Sinai school of medicine complete book of nutrition*, ed. V. Herbert and G. J. Subak-Sharpe, 396-414. New York, NY: St. Martin's Press.

Mannie, K. 1996. *Michigan state football summer conditioning manual*. East Lansing, MI: Michigan State University.

_____. 1988. Key factors in program organization. *High Intensity Training Newsletter 1* (1): 4-5.

_____. 1990. Strength training follies: The all-P.U.B. team. *High Intensity Training Newsletter 2* (2): 11-12.

_____. 1993. Lift risks are a weighty matter. *NCAA News* 30 (January 27): 4-5.

_____. 1994. Some thoughts on explosive weight training. *High Intensity Training Newsletter 5* (1 & 2): 13-18.

Margaria, R., P. Aghemo and E. Rovelli. 1966. Measurement of muscular power (anaerobic) in man. *Journal of Applied Physiology* 21: 1662-1664.

Mayhew, J. L., Prinster, J. L., Ware, J. S., Zimmer, D. L., Arabas, J. R. and M. G. Bemben. 1995. Muscular endurance repetitions to predict bench press strength in men of different training levels. *Journal of Sports Medicine and Physical Fitness* 35 (June): 108-113.

McArdle, W. D., F. I. Katch and V. L. Katch. 1986. *Exercise physiology: Energy, nutrition and human performance*. 2d ed. Philadelphia: Lea & Febiger.

McCarthy, P. 1989. How much protein do athletes really need? *The Physician and Sportsmedicine* 17 (5): 170-175.

Melanson, E. L., P. S. Freedson, R. Webb, S. Jungbluth and N. Kozlowski. 1996. Exercise responses to running and in-line skating at self-selected paces. *Medicine and Science in Sports and Exercise* 28 (February): 247-250.

Mentzer, M. 1993. *Heavy duty*. Venice, CA: Mike Mentzer.

Messier, S. P., and M. Dill. 1985. Alterations in strength and maximal oxygen uptake consequent to Nautilus circuit weight training. *Research Quarterly for Exercise and Sport* 56: 345-351.

Moritani, T., and H. A. deVries. 1979. Neural factors vs hypertrophy in the course of muscle strength gain. *American Journal of Physical Medicine and Rehabilitation* 58: 115-130.

Morton, C. 1990. The relationship between sprint training and conditioning: A time for quality and a time for quantity. *High Intensity Training Newsletter* 2 (3): 9-11.

National Collegiate Athletic Association [NCAA]. 1991. No miracles found in many "natural potions." *NCAA News* 28 (July 17): 7.

NCAA Committee on Competitive Safeguards and Medical Aspects of Sports. 1992. *Ergogenic aids and nutrition*. Overland Park, KS: NCAA memorandum (August 6).

Peterson, J. A., ed. 1978. *Total fitness: The Nautilus way*. West Point, NY: Leisure Press.

_____. 1975. Total conditioning: A case study. *Athletic Journal* 56 (September): 40-55.

Peterson, J. A., and C. X. Bryant, eds. 1992. *The Stairmaster fitness handbook*. Indianapolis: Masters Press.

Peterson, J. A., and C. X. Bryant, eds. 1995. *The Stairmaster fitness hand-book*. 2d ed. St. Louis: Wellness Bookshelf.

Peterson, J. A., and W. L. Westcott. 1990. Stronger by the minute. *Fitness Management* 6 (June): 22-24.

Pezullo, D., S. Whitney and J. Irrgang. 1993. A comparison of vertical jump enhancement using plyometrics and strength footwear shoes versus plyometrics alone. *Journal of Orthopaedic and Sports Physical Therapy* 17: 68.

Piehl, K. 1974. Glycogen storage and depletion in human skeletal muscle fibers. *Acta Physiologica Scandinavica* (Supplementum 402): 1-32.

Pipes, T. V. 1989. *The steroid alternative*. Placerville, CA: Sierra Gold Graphics.

_____. 1979. High intensity, not high speed. *Athletic Journal* 59 (December): 60, 62.

_____. 1988. A.C.T. - The steroid alternative. *Scholastic Coach* 57 (January): 106, 108-109, 112.

_____. 1994. Strength training & fiber types. *Scholastic Coach* 63 (March): 67-70.

Pitts, E. H. 1992. Pills, powders, potions and persuasions. *Fitness Management* 9 (November): 34-35.

Pollock, M. L. 1973. The quantification of endurance training programs. In *Exercise and sports sciences reviews*, ed. J. H. Wilmore, 155-188. New York, NY: Academic Press.

Pollock, M. L., J. Dimmick, H. S. Miller, Z. Kendrick and A. C. Linnerud. 1975. Effects of mode of training on cardiovascular function and body composition of middle-aged men. *Medicine and Science in Sports and Exercise* 7: 139-145.

Porcari, J. P. 1994. Fat-burning exercise: Fit or farce. *Fitness Management* 10 (July): 40-41.

Porcari, J. and J. Curtis. 1996. Can you work strength and aerobics at the same time? *Fitness Management* 12 (June): 26-29.

Rasch, P. J. 1989. *Kinesiology and applied anatomy*. 7th ed. Philadelphia, PA: Lea & Febiger.

Reid, C. M., R. A. Yeater and I. H. Ullrich. 1987. Weight training and strength, cardiorespiratory functioning and body composition in men. *British Journal of Sports Medicine* 21: 40-44.

Reinebold, J. 1993. H.I.T. in the CFL British Columbia style. *High Intensity Training Newsletter* 4 (4): 7-8.

Riley, D. P. 1982. *Strength training by the experts*. 2d ed. West Point, NY: Leisure Press.

_____. 1996. *Redskin conditioning manual*. Ashburn, VA: Washington Redskins.

_____. 1979. Speed of exercise versus speed of movement. *Scholastic Coach* 48 (May/June): 90, 92-93, 97-98.

_____. 1980. Time and intensity: Keys to maximum strength gains. *Scholastic Coach* 50 (November): 65-66, 74-75.

_____. 1982. Guidelines for strength program. *Scholastic Coach* 51 (May/June): 64-65, 80.

Roberts, D. F. 1984. Genetic determinants of sports performance. In *Sport and human genetics*, ed. R. M. Malina and C. Bouchard, 105-121. Champaign, IL: Human Kinetics Publishers, Inc.

Sale, D. G. 1988. Neural adaptation to resistance training. *Medicine and Science in Sports and Exercise* 20: 135-145.

Sale, D. G., and D. MacDougall. 1981. Specificity in strength training: A review for the coach and athlete. *Canadian Journal of Applied Sport Sciences* 6: 87-92.

Saltin, B., J. Henriksson, E. Nygaard and P. Andersen. 1977. Fiber types and metabolic potentials of skeletal muscles in sedentary men and endurance runners. In *The marathon*, ed. P. Milvy. New York: New York Academy of Sciences.

Sargent, V. J. 1921. The physical test of man. *American Physical Education Review* 26 (April): 188-194.

Schantz, P., E. Randall-Fox, W. Hutchison, A. Tyden and P.-O. Astrand. 1983. Muscle fiber type distribution, muscle cross-sectional area and maximal voluntary strength in humans. *Acta Physiologica Scandinavica* 117: 219-226.

Scrimshaw, N. S., and V. R. Young. 1976. The requirements of human nutrition. *Scientific American* 235 (3): 50-64.

Sharkey, B. J. 1975. *Physiology and physical activity.* New York: Harper & Row.

_____. 1984. *Physiology of fitness.* Champaign, IL: Human Kinetics Publishers, Inc.

Singh, A., F. M. Moses and P. A. Deuster. 1992. Chronic multivitamin-mineral supplementation does not enhance physical performance. *Medicine and Science in Sports and Exercise* 24: 726-732.

Skinner, J. S. 1995. Understanding the physiological basis of cardiorespiratory fitness. In *The Stairmaster fitness handbook*, 2d ed, ed. J. A. Peterson and C. X. Bryant, 57-65. St. Louis: Wellness Bookshelf.

Skinner, J. S., and T. McLellan. 1980. The transition from aerobic to anaerobic metabolism. *Research Quarterly for Exercise and Sport* 51: 234-248.

Smith, N. J. 1984. Nutrition. In *Sports medicine*, ed. R. H. Strauss, 468-480. Philadelphia: W. B. Saunders Company.

Sparling, P., R. Recker and T. Lambrinides. 1994. Position statement to football players from Cincinnati Bengals Training Staff and nutrition consultant.

Strauss, R. H., ed. 1984. *Sports medicine*. Philadelphia: W. B. Saunders Company.

Stromme, S. B., and H. Skard. 1980. *Physical fitness and fitness testing*. Sandnes, Norway: Jonas Oglaend A.s.

Swanger, T., M. Bradley and S. Murray. 1996. *Army strength & conditioning manual*. West Point, NY: United States Military Academy.

Taylor, M. R. 1993. The dietary supplement debate of 1993: An FDA perspective. Presented at the Federation of American Societies for Experimental Biology Annual Meeting. New Orleans, LA.

Telford, R., E. Catchpole, V. Deakin, A. Hahn and A. Plank. 1992. The effect of 7 to 8 months of vitamin/mineral supplementation on athletic performance. *International Journal of Sports Nutrition* 2: 135-153.

Thomas, J. 1994. *Penn state football strength training summer conditioning manual*. University Park, PA: Penn State University.

Thompson, C. W. 1985. *Manual of structural kinesiology.* 10th ed. St. Louis: Times Mirror/Mosby College Publishing.

Thorstensson, A. 1976. Muscle strength, fiber types and enzyme activities in man. *Acta Physiologica Scandinavica* (Supplementum 443): 1-44.

Thrash, K., and B. Kelly. 1987. Flexibility and strength training. *Journal of Applied Sport Science Research* 1: 74-75.

Vander, A. J., J. H. Sherman and D. S. Luciano. 1975. *Human physiology: The mechanisms of body function.* 2d ed. New York, NY: McGraw-Hill, Inc.

Vanderburgh, P. M., and W. J. Considine. 1995. Assessing health-related & functional fitness. In *The Stairmaster fitness handbook*, 2d ed, ed. J. A. Peterson and C. X. Bryant, 131-156. St. Louis: Wellness Bookshelf.

Weight, L. M., T. D. Noakes, D. Labadorios, J. Graves, D. Haem, P. Jacobs and P. Berman. 1988. Vitamin and mineral status of trained athletes including the effects of supplementation. *American Journal of Clinical Nutrition* 47: 186-191.

Wells, C. L. 1985. *Women, sport and performance: A physiological perspective.* Champaign, IL: Human Kinetics Publishers, Inc.

Wenger, H. A., and G. J. Bell. 1986. The interactions of intensity, frequency and duration of exercise training in altering cardiorespiratory fitness. *Sports Medicine* 3: 346-356.

Westcott, W. L. 1983. *Strength fitness: Physiological principles and training techniques.* Expanded ed. Boston: Allyn and Bacon, Inc.

_____. 1996. *Building strength and stamina: New Nautilus training for total fitness.* Champaign, IL: Human Kinetics.

_____. 1986. Integration of strength, endurance and skill training. *Scholastic Coach* 55 (May/June): 74.

_____. 1989. Strength training research: sets and repetitions. *Scholastic Coach* 58 (May/June): 98-100.

Wetzel, S. 1994. Letter to the author from the Minnesota Vikings' strength coach. (September 14).

Williams, M. H. 1992. *Nutrition for fitness and sport.* Dubuque, IA: Brown & Benchmark.

Wilmore, J. H. 1982. *Training for sport and activity: The physiological basis of the conditioning process.* 2d ed. Boston: Allyn and Bacon, Inc.

Winett, R. A. 1996. Dose-response. *Master Trainer* 6 (June): 1-2.

Winter, D. A. 1990. *The biomechanics of human movement.* New York, NY: Wiley & Sons.

Wirhed, R. 1984. *Athletic ability: The anatomy of winning.* New York: Harmony Books.

Wolf, M. D. 1982. Muscles: Structure, function and control. In *Strength training by the experts*, 2d ed, by D. P. Riley, 27-40. West Point, NY: Leisure Press.

Wood, K. 1991. Cincinnati Bengals' strength training program. *American Fitness Quarterly* 10 (July): 38, 40.

About the Author

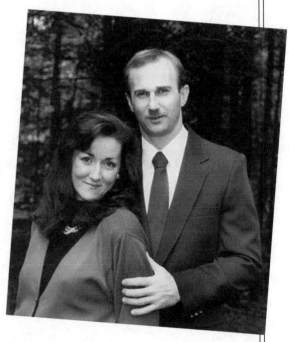

Matt Brzycki received his Bachelor of Science degree in Health and Physical Education from the Pennsylvania State University in 1983. He represented the university for two years in Pennsylvania State Collegiate Powerlifting Championships and was also a place-winner in his first bodybuilding competition. Brzycki served as a health fitness supervisor at Princeton University (NJ) from 1983-84. From 1984-90, he was the Assistant Strength Coach at Rutgers University (NJ). In 1990, he returned to Princeton University as the school's Strength Coach and Health Fitness Coordinator. He was named the Coordinator of Health Fitness, Strength and Conditioning Programs in 1994. Brzycki also teaches a variety of strength and fitness classes for the students, faculty and staff at the university. He developed the Strength Training Theory and Applications course for exercise science and sports studies majors at Rutgers University and has taught the program since March 1990 as a member of the Faculty of Arts and Sciences. He has also taught the same course at The College of New Jersey since 1996.

Brzycki has been a featured speaker at local, regional, state and national conferences and clinics throughout the United States (in CT, IL, KY, LA, MN,

Above: Alicia and Matt Brzycki (photo by Audrey Grimaldi)

NJ, NY, OH, PA and VA) and Canada. He has authored nearly 150 articles that have been featured in more than two dozen different publications. Brzycki has written two other books — *A Practical Approach to Strength Training* and *Youth Strength and Conditioning* — and co-authored *Conditioning for Basketball* with Shaun Brown of the University of Kentucky. (All books published by Masters Press.)

Prior to attending college, Brzycki served in the U. S. Marine Corps from 1975-79 which included a tour of duty as a drill instructor. Among his many responsibilities as a drill instructor was the physical preparedness of Marine recruits. He and his wife, Alicia, currently reside in Lawrenceville, New Jersey, with their child.

Other Masters Press books by Matt Brzycki:

A Practical Approach to Strength Training (3d edition)

Youth Strength and Conditioning

Conditioning for Basketball (with Shaun Brown/University of Kentucky)